Planned UnParenthood

Creating a Life Without Procreating

William (Dann) Alexander

©2012 and ©2015 William (Dann) Alexander
Frogsong Productions
ISBN 978-0-9881486-0-4

William (Dann) Alexander: Planned UnParenthood

Table of Contents

Foreword

My wife and I were new owners of a "just married" sign the previous August. We had decided it was time to expand our family. I will never forget the day we brought the twins home for the first time. Everything had been finalized. The adoption went through with absolutely no delays.

It was a short drive home from where we picked them up and everything was ready to go. We were well prepared. We bought a fair supply of baby food and owned everything we needed to keep them warm for the approaching winter cold. These are the times where you learn to quickly appreciate the discounts available in big box department stores.

We were going to be permitted to give the kids names. My wife decided right away they would be Leonard and Stanley. They are not named after anyone in particular. However, this has not stopped my mother from telling her friends and work colleagues that they are named after Canadian singer/songwriters Leonard Cohen and Stan Rogers.

To this day, I am amazed at how much the twins look like their biological parents. Stanley looks like his mom, while Leo looks like his Dad. The resemblances were astounding. We even met the parents just as we finalized the adoption paperwork.

The Mom was a bit apprehensive with us at first, while it seemed like the Dad was very content. He must have sensed that his kids would be going to a good home where they would be well looked after. This gave me great peace of mind. In an adoption process where the biological parents are involved, it is good knowing that as the adopting family, you have the parents' approval.

When we introduced the boys to their sisters, there was a bit of hesitation on behalf of our oldest girl, who had turned eight a few months prior. It has since taken her four years just getting used to them being around. Our second oldest girl seemed to not mind them at all. She would walk up to them and check them out, never saying a word. She would not try to play with them since they were just infants, but at least she was genuinely pleasant with them overall.

From the start, Leo was a very happy –go-lucky kid. He was instantly finding great joy in the simple things. It seems to take little to nothing in order to make him happy.

Stanley seems to be a bit clingy, although the way he sticks to us is very loving. He loves to be held and that seems to be his greatest joy. Usually he prefers to snuggle with his Mom since she showers them both with the most attention. She also spent the most time with both dogs in the days after they first arrived home so the bond was much stronger for her.

I chalked up my oldest girl's issues of jealousy as being a case of classic sibling rivalry. Most parents have a genuine understanding of this process and how it works amongst their children. It can be difficult to manage at times for most. Few times I will hear parents talk about how their children never fight amongst themselves or never get along with each other. Those seem to be rare instances.

In late July of 2007, we welcomed a new addition whom we named Olive into the family, making the number of children a healthy and busy five. It was another successful adoption. We know we must be doing something right with our children when we realized we could leave them for a few hours completely on our own without worry.

But cats are like that. It just so happens that the twins will require more attention. As dogs, they need someone with them on a regular basis because they require more attention.

There is a seemingly quiet, but rapidly building global community of individuals who are speaking out about the decision to not birth children. In writing this book, one of the goals is to educate others about why people come to this decision.

Perhaps for some of you, several questions will be created and even answered in the pages that follow the questions. Being childfree is not a philosophy based on a set of decisions. Rather, it is about choosing a lifestyle for a variety of reasons.

In speaking with so many people about this idea and through a significant amount of research, I have been fortunate in obtaining a plethora of viewpoints on how people react to someone who says they don't want children.

Not wanting children is accepted by most as a matter of personal choice. However, childfreedom is rapidly ridiculed by others based on different beliefs. Some people of strong, (and dare I say it) extremist religious backgrounds vehemently oppose the idea that people can go out of their way not to have children. Many of those people will impose religious belief on childfree people insisting that having children is a "decision up to God".

As people we have the power to make choices, and part of making those choices is living with any consequences of those choices.

Let's face it; freedom of choice is one of the most taken for granted constitutional gifts in a democracy. When a person decides not to have children, regardless of what other people think, it should be a celebration of choice. It is not an open door for launching a vicious attack on someone's personal life.

You may have picked up this book because you are contemplating the decision whether or not to have children. Maybe you are a fence-sitter watching people on both sides of that fence while you mull over the choice.

As you check the view from the place you are sitting, you will see me amongst the people on the side where people have concluded to have zero children. With all confidence, I am proud to state that my life is better for having made this decision. It has been easy for me to accept the negatively perceived "consequences" of making this choice.

Society's negative perceptions of those who are childfree are narrowly focused opinions meant to put people on some low rung of a human ladder of importance.

Many will accuse childfree people of having a lack of knowledge with respect to the "joys" of having children. Inclusion of this ridiculous interrogative is the suggestion that there is the potential for becoming a better person by having children. We are often told that somehow childfree are "missing out" on these supposed joys.

Mind you, these are often the same people who go into parenthood with the same alleged lack of knowledge. Or, they will be the ones who dispense parental advice with "you just have to do it" as the answer to every question from other parents. In response to missing out on the joys of having children, I reply that for me the joys of childfreedom far outweigh any responsibility that I would want as a parent.

I will also acknowledge a group of people who are often largely forgotten when speaking of families; the empty nesters. Empty nesters have grown children that have moved out of the house. You will see as I go further in these pages, that empty nesters should also receive the same treatment as those who are childfree.

Later in these pages, you will note that some of my ideas for fairness towards childfree families are also geared towards those who for whatever reason cannot have children.

Much of the world fails to understand the childfree lifestyle and writes it off as some sort of evil ignorant thinking. People with close-minded opinions on childfreedom are not even willing to entertain the opinions of the global childfree community.

People may read words in childfree reasoning that will open their eyes further to good ideas. In these instances, a few readers will find things that will provoke more thought and debate.

I know that the pages following will inspire, enlighten and perhaps enrage.

So enjoy.

Sincerely,

William (Dann) Alexander

Chapter 1

The Precision of a Decision

Life is full of choices and results from those choices. We get a daily dose of decision making on things from what to have for breakfast to whether we will tackle house-cleaning today, tomorrow or a week from now.

Then there are always the big major decisions which can have a lasting impact on our lives. Pondering these decisions is akin to flying on a commercial passenger jet. Making the decision on whether to have children can be the equivalent of a long flight overseas to new lands unknown. Deciding to not have children is hardly a one hour commuter flight.

The turbulence on the flight is a trip through a heavy cloud of weighing the consequences and any family and peer pressures you may be faced with.

If you make the decision with confidence, you are descending back to ground level, focused and confident on your life direction. Some people will leave the option open of flying again to review and evaluate the choice. It is a proven fact that a few who are leaning towards being childfree may change that decision mid-flight.

Most who have confidently decided on childfreedom come into a perfect landing and walk into arrivals, knowing they have made a choice that they feel is right. They grab the luggage full of consequences and walk out, heading back into the busy world enveloping them.

I am unable to pinpoint the exact time where I walked into the arrivals area of this decision. What I am fairly certain of is that my decision was made with a high level of self-assurance, and I have not wavered on this choice since.

It was sometime between the last year of elementary school and my seventh grade year when I became more certain of my childfree intent.

I once read a statement while conducting some research that said, "Biology is not Destiny". This sentence has since become a rallying cry for those who have chosen not to have children. I was so moved by reading this that I placed it as the wallpaper on my computer desktop while in college. It is a rebellion against the ill-conceived impression that we as humans are all brought to life on earth specifically to conceive and populate the planet.

I am of the longstanding belief that regardless of what I do, who I am and who I become, I am here to *live.*

Part of that living is making personal choices and exercising personal freedoms. My functioning brain cells concluded a long time ago that I was more than capable of knowing right from wrong, based on learning.

It is up to me to make the most of life. Having no children is one of the best decisions I ever made. It hardly makes me ignorant of the joys of life. If anything, it has given me more awareness of the abundance I have.

Parents to me always seem to have the busier lives and never appear to have time to themselves. My life was going to be busy enough with all of the passions and pursuits I intended to follow. Parenting would be a major sacrifice of personal space and time. I was and am still not prepared to sacrifice my personal and professional time to be Dad to any human children.

Most parents I have met in my travels seemed to constantly be giving up their own dreams (albeit honourably), in order to live up to the responsibilities of parenthood.

How often has anyone heard tale of a parent who had aspirations to be this or that, but put it all aside to raise children? Some of these parents then go on a minute-long speaking spree to quickly defend their decision. With a few parents who are giving these defensive sounding speeches, it is almost like they are talking in order to cover up any element of regret they may feel.

I have great respect for parents who have privately admitted to me that they regret having children, but instead of living in that regret, they have turned their energy to being the best parent they can be. I have always hoped that this kind of strategy may work to perhaps change their regret.

The way I envisioned my future life was just not in line with that of a parent. I know my own parents were busy enough people and it seemed like they had minimal time for their personal pursuits.

I can enter a plea of guilty for outright lying at one point in time, pretending to want children in order to look good to someone else. I felt a tremendous sense of guilt for temporarily not being true to myself. Underneath the lie, I never once intended to change course on this decision.

Although I may not have ever wanted to be the "parent" of children, what I wanted is to be a responsible and loving "parent" to animals.

My Grandmother's dedication to the care and love for animals influenced me from a very young age. She was a passionate and caring woman whom at her best health would have rescued every animal if she could. If only she had the space and financial resources. I share her sentiments today. Some people may easily identity with this feeling. You may be a loving and caring parent of a "fur baby". Anyone falling under that category will often refer to their pets as "children".

It is remarkably sad that some people cannot understand that a person can love an animal just as much, if not more, than they would a child. In a world where aggravated mistrust can alter one's view on humankind, it is understandable that some people have much more faith in the animal kingdom.

When asked if we have any children and knowing full well they mean human children, I love to see the look on people's faces when we reply. "My wife and I have five children, and want many more."

My Grandmother would be proud of how well looked after our "children" are. She supported my decision not to have children and never once questioned why I felt so strongly.

Sitting down over tea and sandwiches I would just say to her in a matter-of-fact tone, "Gram, I am not going to have children". To which she would reply "Okay! Have some tea". I figure the world does not need another one of me filling up notebooks with words, leaving them in different places of a house.....

As a young teen, I was becoming more aware of my decision to not have children that I began sharing my views with others. Be it teachers, classmates, friends, family and whoever would listen. I remember hearing conversations among some of the girls about what they would name their kids one day, how many they wanted to have and other things along that line of thinking. Plus, I would hear varying stories about how they would go about parenting their children.

I would witness first-hand a few of those classmates and some friends put themselves through the turbulence of teenage pregnancy. With that sudden life transition you have young teens who have to become responsible adults overnight. Suddenly a few people in nearby desks were balancing parenthood with school, living life with a whole different perspective.

Responsibility takes on a whole new meaning when someone is expecting a child. Classmates who became parents at a young age immediately gave themselves much more responsibility instantaneously.

It was also during that time in junior high school that I made a bet with myself. It would mark a significant part of my life where I would eventually take the step to ensure I never could become a parent.

I began to read about the vasectomy right around the time I was an observer to some classmates who were about to become parents. My Grandparents kept this weird book in their living room which described about every surgery you could imagine. This book contained detailed descriptions of surgical procedures, with crudely drawn computer images of each surgery.

For most men the thought of a needle or knife coming anywhere near their member sends a shiver of disgust through their spinal columns.

The vasectomy remains a popular elective among men who wish to ensure they have no further children, or in my case have no children at all.

I made a bet with myself that I would have the operation before I turned twenty-five. I was set and stubborn. This was going to happen, regardless of where I ended up in life or where it took me. In the early part of 2002 at the age of twenty-three, I met with my family physician to seek the necessary referral to a urologist.

That appointment is still vividly memorable. Somehow I managed to remain calm and even explained "the bet" to him. The good doctor listened to me for about two minutes before sitting down in a nearby chair.

He paused for a moment, wiping the sweat from his forehead and asked, "Do you want to see a psychiatrist first?" This took me by complete surprise. Although I was surprised to see his head shaking, it was a major relief that he agreed to the referral. He must have realized I was legitimate in my thinking.

For several months leading up to the procedure, the amount of criticism I received mounted. This was mostly from people well outside of my own close circle of friends and family.

Few of my friends ever questioned my decision since they have known all along how I felt. "What if you change your mind?" won the award for most common question put forth.

The most disturbing criticism I did receive were comments from a religious fanatic who somehow thought I was doomed for a life in hell since I was going to manipulate my body in a "negative" way. How negative is a vasectomy, really? If science has advanced to a point where an operation like this is available, men have every right to take advantage of such a procedure.

I fail to see how making this decision is a negative thing. Some men may change their mind later in life. They might decide they want to have children the natural way.

Medicine has also advanced to such a progressive stage where a vasectomy reversal can be performed. The success rates for these reversals vary depending on a large number of biological factors of each man.

So, at the age of twenty-three in the late fall of 2002, I made good on the bet. I took the step of ensuring I could never become a parent naturally. I waited until after the operation to let my family know what I had done. To my surprise, the majority of them were tremendously supportive and understanding. The backlash was minimal.

My main reason for not wanting to have children was briefly outlined in previous pages. Parents seem to just have insanely busy lives with little time for anything else.

I and many others are not prepared to make this kind of lifetime commitment knowing it will take up so much time and energy. To me, the time sacrifice is just simply not worth it. I have elected to use that time in the efforts of pursuing my life passions and directing any parental instincts towards providing a good life for animals, my supportive spouse, and myself.

There are a myriad of other reasons why others will choose no children. Many people might fear that they could come to resent parenthood later. A person does not have children with the intent that they may resent them, but the fear of that potential resentment definitely could be a factor. This might be viewed as a form of the parent trap.

Having children may build an immediate bar of restriction on lifestyle options a family may want to undertake. If children are suddenly in the picture, then opportunities to travel may become limited. Friends and other extended family may want to set a date and time for a trip or activity, but they may pass on contacting them automatically assuming that they will be too busy with their children.

Many fence-sitters have told me they may also be fearful of passing on any existing medical conditions to children they could have. Many ailments that are theoretically manageable in day-to-day living may be still incredibly consuming in one's life. That person may fear having a kid who could end up with the same ailment.

Like any decisions there will always be consequences. Those choosing no children will argue strongly that there are many more potential consequences for having them. For fence-sitters, know that you need to educate yourself as much as possible and look at both sides before choosing whether to conceive.

Chapter 2

Just Say No to Midnight Feedings

In 2001, a Statistics Canada study found that out of 24,000 people interviewed, eight percent of men and seven percent of women planned to be childfree by choice. The reasons for making this decision vary, yet are common among many childfree families.

For some, the presence of children in a social situation may cause great anxiety and stress. Fact is that children require supervision. Therefore, someone may not feel comfortable in a social situation where the supervising adult may suddenly leave the room.

Suddenly that person may become the acting supervisor! For a brief few seconds, or minutes, you could be the sole person completely responsible for that child even if no one charges you with the duty of watching the kid. Most childfree people that openly admit to not liking kids may never allow themselves to be put into this situation anyways.

Those that do end up watching kids in that situation may feel an immediate anxiety.

Here they are, suddenly for a few minutes as the one person in the room who can prevent that child from hurting themselves. They do not want to be held responsible for the child if something were to happen to them.

Every parent has to face those moments of children falling on the floors, bumping their heads on tables, or any other number of hopefully minor accidents around the home. If the child is hurt for some reason as a result of those accidents, it is probably the parent they will want comfort from first. They will not necessarily run to the friend or relative in the room.

Then there are people who do not like children and freely admit to this. Seems like a good reason not to have children! Surely there would be universal agreement that someone who does not like kids should just not have them.

I have only been recently made aware of the term paedophobia, which is defined as an absolute fear of infants and children. This is an actual diagnosis that psychiatrists have given to people. What is somewhat alarming is that there are parents who have been diagnosed with this very fear!

Some parents who are diagnosed with paedophobia are more likely to be afraid of any children and infants but their own. I have read that a fear of infants may manifest as a result of a person's inability to comprehend them.

It is a major misconception among people that all childfree people dislike children. Just because someone doesn't want them, doesn't mean they don't like them.

I have moved tables at restaurants and movie theatres to get away from children whose parents were doing nothing to quiet them down and make them behave properly. Never should anyone have to put up with the awkwardness crafted from of this kind of scenario. For the longest time I was afraid to act in these situations. Once I finally had enough courage to move from that table or switch rows, it became easier to stand my ground.

The time where I started to become more aware about being in these situations was a painfully long flight in 1999. In two of the seats ahead of me was a young father with his toddler son. This kid was up on his seat every five minutes. He spent the majority of the flight looking around the plane cabin or waving his hands in my face for what seemed like an eternity.

The young father, who was probably not much older than me, was exercising some phony discipline just turning his kid around and sitting him back down without a word of stern discipline.

Finally more than three quarters of the way into the flight, the kid was silenced to sleep. He had fallen asleep from his constant movement. Now since this was pre-911, we were still in a time where flight attendants brought children up to the cockpit where they received a hello from the captain and first officer. This trip to the front would make the visiting children honorary pilots. The stewardess went to bring this young kid but thankfully the father insisted on letting him sleep. My patience had long run out at that point so I was delighted that the remainder of the flight would continue in peace.

Some people genuinely crave peace and quiet of a less populated household. Choosing to have children reduces and, in some cases, eliminates that constant quiet. Parenthood is a major responsibility that requires one to be alert and aware almost constantly. I am often hearing friends and family who are complaining of a lack of sleep and time for themselves. They are tired from the daily grind that parenthood provides.

Ultimately, I acknowledge that a parent needs to find that positive balance. Families where children are present come home needing to focus all of their energy towards how their kids' day went, if they have homework, how daycare was for the younger ones, among an avalanche of things that just have to be acknowledged. Then there is ensuring a meal is prepared and the kitchen cleaned up after. All of the daily tasks seem to multiply in detail when kids are around.

Of course there might be a bona-fide battle with one kid who does not like what is put in front of them at the dinner table. Surely each of you reading this loathed one food or another that your parents made you eat.

Once supper is done and the dishes are cleaned up, there might be extra-curricular activities that evening if they are not already started right after school is out. Perhaps some sport that the parent wishes they had excelled in when they were young.

Do not forget piano lessons for the son who wants to grow his hair long and play loud music. Then at some point the kids all have to go to bed and actually stay in it. By the time everything settles down, you look at your significant other and wish you had enough strength to finally speak a private sentence, or the stamina to share a moment of intimacy, but you fall asleep dead tired, as it is well past midnight.

To add to any perceived craziness, a newborn infant needs to be fed throughout the day and into the night. This means the possibility of midnight and 4 a.m. feedings!

No thanks! I really value my sleep. In my universe every second of rest counts. I could not even imagine the idea of having to get up in the middle of the night to the sound of a child crying into some cheap one-way radio. All of the technology that has developed over the years for these radios should have been spent on creating a Baby Babble Translator.

I would much prefer to be woken up by my dogs telling me they need to go outdoors or to check out something a cat may have knocked over than get up during the night every four hours to feed an infant.

I know, not every single family scenario plays out like this. The illustration that I have painted is an example of something happening somewhere in this world as you read this. Every family is different. Every child is different. Every set schedule in every household is different.

As a kid and through my teens, I kept a small yet close circle of friends. I also spent a ton of time doing stuff on my own enjoying peaceful quiet time. Friends who came by would find me reading, playing video games, outside at a nearby basketball court, writing or cranking out loud music. Once I earned the privilege of driving, I took to the open road quite frequently as a form of relaxation.

I have always favoured going for drives out to rural areas or often-forgotten tourist attractions as a form of alert meditation. I preferred to relish the quiet time when and where

I could find it. Having children would in my view, take much of that down time away.

Most people will agree that parenthood is a lifetime commitment. Bringing a child into the world should be a commitment to doing the best you can to raise them well. With that commitment naturally a significant amount of stress may be attracted. I constantly hear parents of perceived "good" children all the time talk about how they never stress out about their kids. Anyone who tells you they never worry about their children is committing self-deception. Some of these parents may exercise great patience on the outside, yet within them is a pounding heart and heavy head worrying about the slightest things.

I believed the old television station and radio airwave message "It's 11:00, do you know where your children are?" was meant to trigger anxiety and panic attacks in every parent.

It must have worked well. We do not see or hear those messages anymore. This is likely due to a volume of complaints from therapists who accused the media of enabling madness. A parent somewhere right now is worrying about their teenager getting home on time within their imposed curfew. If that kid comes in one minute past curfew then the parent must exercise the rules of household law enforcement. This is the ever-evolving exercise of discipline.

The idea of having to create and enforce discipline can easily be credited as another reason for childfree people to make the choices they have made. Parenting is a lot of work. Discipline can make up a significant portion of that work.

There are so many different ways to address and talk about discipline that I have given it an entire chapter later on. This is one of the defining reasons childfree people do not want the worry nor do they want to even remotely think about enforcement.

There is another D word which is another major reason why some people will not have children. Diapers! Bowel and urinary functions are not taboo subjects anymore. But there are people who do not want to have to clean up after anyone else but themselves.

We can now pick up celebrity gossip rags and once in a while read details about the bodily functions of celebrity offspring.

Some people believe this normal function of life somehow is the biggest control factor in their kids' lives. I remember a television interview where a certain singer who should have been talking about her new record instead spent more than a few dreadful sentences talking about how it was all about the shit. No literally, I mean the actual shit. Well at least I could change the channel.

I also remember watching an interview of one of my favorite

actresses talk about her infant son and how she made up a song about how amazed she was at a shit-filled diaper. That's right! A song!

She could have parlayed that talent into re-writing some dialogue in a bad movie she did.

I am fairly certain that most people do not find the smell of shit even the slightest bit appealing. If you do, I advise you to seek help.

There was one particular time in a medical office where I witnessed a nauseating parental task.

I was waiting in my chiropractor's office for an appointment. A young father was wrestling to keep his infant son from running all over the office. This kid was wearing a diaper that stuck halfway out of his pants. The young and obviously tired father quietly asked his kid in toddler-friendly language if he had gone to the bathroom. He then picked him up, pulled back his son's pants and took a disturbingly long sniff. His face soured before swiftly making a beeline for the washroom with son in tow.

I was repulsed and revolted. It dawned on me that for probably a long time during a kid's early years this could have been one of the daily tasks I would be sharing with my spouse. In this very short yet memorable visit to the chiropractor's office, I managed to receive a generous reminder of one of the many reasons to elect childfreedom.

Travelling with children also adds a significant amount of work to the task of getting places. Long road trips require many bathroom breaks and possibly more stops to eat and get supplies. Whereas between me, my wife and some animals, we have very quick breaks and are on our way. We are able to make efficient use of our break time and resume the journey.

With children, there will be additional factors that may require parents to stop their vehicles more for the children. It is probably difficult for driving parents to sometimes deal with the temper tantrums that might happen. If it escalates to the point of a meltdown, then pulling over to the side of the road might be in order to gain control of the situation.

Meltdowns have to be averted somehow! The threat of "turning this car around and going home" is still the universal attempt to avert a meltdown or sibling fight in a vehicle.

If you have travelled at all, you might have witnessed a situation when it comes to children and airline travel. Families with children have to organize and plan ahead when it comes to moving through the skies. Families with maybe three or four children that end up travelling on an aircraft have to hope they will find enough seats together.

Many times I have seen parents having to sit in two seats while across the aisle the three children they have need to have all kinds of toys, food and everything else that will distract them and help pass time during the flight.

In the few instances where I have come across this situation, most of the parents have been very responsible. In the handful of occasions where the situation was unpleasant, moving seats could be an option. Also, thanks to the increase in available entertainment on flights, the volume on the television or radio can be turned up loud to drown out any such craziness if it happens.

A significant amount of financial resources are needed in the raising and care of children. In North America, raising a child to the age of eighteen will cost anywhere from thirty-thousand to over three-hundred thousand dollars. There are many internet sites that offer some sort of perspective on costs where they are factoring in different circumstances.

My own personal view is that the three-hundred thousand dollar tag might be very realistic. This is especially true if a parent is planning to send their child to higher learning.

I am happy to pay my bills and buy food, and provide care for my beloved pets. I do not want to have to put more food in the fridge for more than two people, save for maybe extra for a night of entertaining. Nor do I wish to have to save money for a child's college fund. That is money I can spend elsewhere, like buying my wife some new shoes!

Childfree people will usually have more disposable income than an average family with children. If a family with kids and a family without children is paying their bills on time and has equal debt, then of course the family without children has more money on hand at the end of the day.

Many of the motivating factors in having no children revolve around giving themselves more of what they need. Fact is people need time for themselves and their personal interests. Parents who are able to find alone time and raise good kids are to be saluted. Some people have developed a balanced method or two where they factor this time in to pursue interests.

People who schedule this personal time are more bound to ensure they get that moment or two of solitude.

Many parents neglect their own health whilst participating in the day to day regime parenthood commands of them. Chasing after children could be considered a workout on its own.

However, I do not believe this to be the most effective or consistent way to exercise. Whether it is a sport you like or a walk in the park, proper exercise and relaxation are keys to living healthy. There is little doubt that many parents struggle to find that balance.

Instead of spending even a remote amount of time looking after themselves, many parents find they end up in chauffeur roles once they are clear of the work day.

They go from working parental support to taxi driver just so their children can attend events the parents wished they had excelled at in younger days. It is admirable that many of the hockey dads and soccer moms are so devoted to having their children involved in things. But I believe more children should discover those things on their own. If they show an interest in something positive then it should be pursued.

How many of you as kids were forced into music lessons or sports you may have disliked?

The downfall of pushing kids in activities is that many parents become militant dictators at some of these events. Go and attend any children's hockey or soccer games, and you are guaranteed to find several examples of this kind of draconian parental guidance.

The concept of unschooling free play is where children learn using exploration in recreation. If kids are involved in a sport or activity they want to be in, then surely they have the basics of the activity formed in their mind.

When they start attending these events, they would have a coach or instructor present to guide them. To apply this to the hockey example, kids who are starting out might be given a large bag of pucks on the ice and left to improvise what happens from there.

Most if not all of those kids will then take the hockey pucks and practice shooting on the net. A few might work on passing or rapid-fire skating with the puck on the stick.

To relate to this further, let me tell you that I am a member of a group of alumni who played hockey for a small town in Nova Scotia. In addition to playing hockey I attended several divisional games where my brother was playing for a more experienced team.

The majority of the time parents were generally supportive of their kids. Those parents were doing, and saying all of the right things. This was a golden era of time when minor hockey rules were significantly strictor. Kids could not even deliver clean on-ice hits to other kids in the name of gaining puck control.

As much as I loved the game as a kid, (and still do now), there was one particular game I attended as an observer that gave me my first insight into the sheer insanity of some parents.

One of the teams my brother and I loathed playing against was nearby Thorburn. We both went to school with many people in the Thorburn organization. It was an insane rivalry. I viewed it as the local equivalent of the classic National Hockey League Toronto Maple Leafs and Montreal Canadiens feud.

It was the only time I would actually train several days before a game. I wanted to win against them so bad that it consumed me. I wanted our team to get more goals, out skate and out play so I could have bragging rights Monday morning at school. It may be one of the few times where playing hockey for fun and the concept of free play almost went right out the door for me.

At a game where my brother's divisional club played Thorburn, a shoving match had erupted between two players. I was wedged in the stands between sets of angry Trenton parents and a group of Thorburn parents who were just as upset. A fine line had been crossed. The referees stepped in to warn the players and teams to calm down and cool off. Back then, you could face immediate suspension for the entire year if you crossed that line.

The game continued but there was more roughness that was escalating. The parental groups started launching into attacks. They were blaming each other's children for the escalation of the unnecessary roughness. Eventually somehow the game went through ending in a 1-0 victory for my brother's club.

I remember also leaving the rink in sheer shock at the lack of maturity in these parents. It was not about ensuring their kids were having fun. It became the war between sets of rival parents whose own dreams failed amidst a sea of winter coats and empty cups of chalk-flavored cocoa.

Many of the parents were positively involved in what their kids were up to. Even in a losing cause, my folks were always quick to emphasize having fun as the most important thing. My Dad was occasionally trying to offer tips and advice for the right reasons. He realized after a while I was not too interested in the mechanics of the game and just wanted to play.

My wife experienced a more recent minor hockey game that reinforced the sad state of minor sports programs for children. Parents were screaming for their children to hit others at the tops of their lungs.

It was as if the parents maybe wanted to see their kids be tough so others would maybe leave them alone. Not just with the game, but with life in general. These were over-caffeinated hockey parents hoping their kids will put them into wealthy early retirement by having them get to the NHL level.

The idea of extra-curricular fun for kids is completely lost on the majority of parents today.

Everyone, and I do mean everyone, knows someone who was pushed into music lessons, or some other kind of artful pursuit at the forced hand of a parent. Like any other extra-curricular activity, parents should want their children to discover artistic pursuits on their own.

There is of course, a major cost to having children in these extra-curricular activities. The cost of having a kid playing minor hockey for example can now run well into the thousands. When you add up the costs of equipment, registration fees, and even fuel to get from game to game and tournament to championship game, that cost could reach even higher.

The same types of comments could be said for other sports naturally. Soccer may cost significantly less in the form of equipment, but there is still the fuel, food and time.

It is hard to ignore the fact that many kids are in sports because their parents force them into it. This is all part of a greater effort to live through their children and have them try and succeed at the parents failed dreams. I have mentioned that in many instances parents have their children enrolled in arts programs for the same reasons.

This all comes back to a summarization. People who have children will often choose to do so at the expense of giving up their personal dreams. Some observers around them will accuse parents of trying to live through their children by pushing them into things the parents wanted to succeed at.

Often, many of these children want nothing to do with these particular things. Whether it is lessons on a musical instrument they won't even touch or taking part in some sport, this often ignorantly serves to please the parent at the expense of making their child downright miserable.

Rarely do I hear tale of kids being involved in things based on their actual interests. When I do hear those tales it is really a positive experience. I have heard many great true parental stories about how their sons and or daughters cannot wait for the coming sports seasons, or how they are performing at an upcoming show/recital/concert.

Children should have a voice on what they want to be involved in. Parents often will not give their children a voice and just force them into the first thing they can think of. I very much believe the same can be said for religion. Children can and should be taught right from wrong, but when it comes to spirituality and faith, they should be taught to think and make choices on their own.

Those without children are also more likely and able to spend time working on their personal relationships. Those relationships could be that of close friendships or existing family and social ties.

Arguably the biggest relationship one can have is the love shared with their significant other. In my view, this is possibly one of the most important relationships one could have.

Those without children are automatically drawn to focus more on that connection. For some couples with children, the intimate times they share becomes few and far between. This can result in significant stress and strain on the whole relationship.

Many parents find themselves too exhausted to have a regularly scheduled date between the sheets. Some American psychologists estimate that between fifteen to twenty percent of couples will have sex no more than ten times a year. What I wondered is what percentage of those couples have children?

In my days of watching too much garbage television, I can remember an episode of a long-gone talk show that was centered on the lack of intimacy in the marriage. In each interview of the subject couples, the chief complaint was that one spouse was always tired because they had to do stuff for their children, all the time, and every time.

Perhaps they were using this as an excuse? Maybe the presence of children is a way for someone in the marriage to hide behind some deeper emotional issues? Or perhaps the stories were the real deal and these couples have given up on any hope of regular intimacy.

In no way am I suggesting that every childfree couple is living a life of frequent sex and a million a day exchanges of affection. I reiterate that those without children are more likely to spend more time on sharing those intimate moments with their partners.

The only midnight feeding I'll gladly take part in is a round of appetizers after ringing in the New Year.

Chapter 3

Natalist Perceptions

Society seems to be born with a natalist view, believing that having children is supposed to be a part of life for everyone.   Social situations for childfree people can be the most common breeding ground for expression of many stereotypical viewpoints.

Let me paint you a scene that repeats itself in syndication among many who have chosen no children.

A childfree couple is at a gathering. It is a semi-formal affair at a fancy banquet room. Drinks flow from the bar. People are mixing it up. The childfree couple is among many making the rounds.

A couple with two, maybe three children approaches, perhaps afraid to admit that they are happy to have a break from their parental responsibilities in order to drink and take a taxi home.

An introduction to spouses follows. The parental units find a query delivered from the warehouse of common social questions. "Have any children?"

Time and space for a brief millisecond, will come to a complete halt. The maternal unit is anticipating childfree man to flip open his faux leather wallet and have several pictures of children fall out for the room to see.

This does not happen. First of all, childfree man owns a velcro vinyl wallet absent pictures of kids, politely replying "No children". The parental units suddenly share a quick glance of stunned amazement before returning to the conversation.

"Really? Well when will you have them?" Childfree woman then tells the parental units proudly that she and her husband will never have children. Within this short period of time, the conversation has gone from exchanging pleasantries to formation and delivery of poor judgment by the parental units. This is a judgment that is still too common in many social situations.

Saying you do not have children, or plan to not have children can be a social bomb. This is only because many people still insist that we are here to conceive and bring forward life.

What I have always found striking in these social situations are the follow-up questions. The most aggravating question to me is "Why would you not have children who can take care of you later?"

Really? This person clearly had other intentions for birthing her kids. This kind of idiotic thinking led me to believe she brought her children into the world for the purpose of training them as personal care workers.

That's career encouragement for you.

When you reflect further on this thinking, this particular woman who asked the question obviously has some fear about no one being there for her when she is older. That is a door to another set of issues this person probably has altogether.

It is up to each of us individually to take care of ourselves so that we live long healthy and prosperous lives.

The fact remains that society as a whole expects people to conceive and birth children. People should want to have children on their own free will.

Television has acted as an open book of tragic stories of couples who for whatever reason, are unable to conceive and have children.

A positive aspect of seeing some of these stories is that medicine has advanced to such a level where the treatment options are becoming more widely available for those considered infertile. Of course with these treatments becoming so mass produced, there are a handful of people who have chosen to abuse these methods in an effort to gain fame.

The darker side of television has given birth to more reality programming for a very small crew of publicity seeking money-starved families. This kind of exploitation has to be the most widely ignored sub-category of child abuse. These types of television shows have eclipsed the number of documented real-life tragedies of people who cannot have children, despite wanting to.

Society's natalist tendency needs to become more open-minded with positive and proactive understanding of the childfree decision. What people choose to do with their lives and how many children they should have, if any, is ultimately one of the most personal choices one will ever make. Influences will have an effect on this choice, be it negative or positive.

A perfect example of the natalist philosophy is the evangelical Christian "Quiverfull" movement. The apparent creed behind

Quiverfull in my opinion depowers women to a mandate of having them just be childrearing homemakers. Quiverfull followers shun any form of birth control and believe having children is a "marked blessing from God."

German Philosopher Arthur Schopenhauer was an advocate of opposition to natalist tendencies. Antinatalism is an ideology advancing the awareness of the potential negatives of having children. In particular, antinatalism provokes thought on how having children could contribute to problems like over-population and strains on government programs in some countries.

Antinatalism, while considered a pessimistic view on the birthing of children, has significant validity weaved amongst its' theoretical threads. Schopenhauer wrote in favour of an antinatalist viewpoint, suggesting in his writings that having children just for the reason of having them was placing a burden on the remainder of society.

Mind you, he wrote this at a time long before public systems of health and daycare existed. Subsequently, we now have systems which are often strained for hospital beds and daycare spaces.

Antinatalism could be viewed as an oppositional standpoint to the peace and love culture of the 60's. Instead of free-loving natalists with a more open-view of the indulgences, antinatalists were giving people insight into a pessimistic side of life on earth.

The most obvious problem with antinatalism is that it is mostly a negative point of view. I understand why people like Schopenhauer felt the way they did, but it is a very pessimistic view.

While I quickly defend the reasons anyone has for not having children, I would say that by no means do I spend time encouraging others never to have them. I always joke that everyone should have children except me. Fact is, I wish only the right people were having children and for the right reasons. If people want to have children in order to have someone look after them when they are older, then they might as well at least be up front with their reasoning.

Let us envision the childfree and parental unit couples at the same social gathering, a few years into the future. This is after a mass public education campaign of respect and understanding regarding the choices.

Maternal unit asks her question again. "Children?" Childfree lady replies calmly but coolly, "We have chosen to have no children". The parental units nod in understanding and acceptance.

Mr. Parental unit then pulls out his faux-leather wallet, allowing the plastic photo holders and their contents to flop out. "Here are my future personal care workers".

Chapter 4

Prejudice

Arguably, the biggest breeding ground of prejudice towards those without children is in the workplace. Companies who claim to be "family friendly" do so to give parents special consideration. Many of these same so called "family friendly" companies however, do not show the same consideration to people without children.

Overwhelmingly, parents are given preferential treatment in any workplace over their childfree (and childless) colleagues. If someone has to be called in for overtime, the bosses are more likely to reach for the phone number of the person without kids.

Even if they live with their spouse, several cats, dogs and maybe even a brilliant parrot that can quote lines from Shakespeare, they are the first ones to be called. Granted, some bosses will call the person who might have infant children, but often out of sympathy in assuming that parents might need some extra cash on their cheque to cover childcare costs.

I would challenge that discrimination against those without children continually runs rampant throughout a majority of workplaces. This would be including these so-called family friendly places.

Those without children are always assumed to be available because many managers assume those people have fewer responsibilities. Most managers forget that the employee without children has a life as well, and may not want to work the overtime.

This type of situation puts the workplace on a very uneven field. It may pit colleagues against each other. Holidays, such as Christmas, are where you can sometimes see the most obvious examples. The rotational on-call person is likely going to be the person with no children.

Most management assumes the person with no children will be ready and willing to work on a holiday. Never mind the person probably was looking forward to a wonderful holiday with their significant other or extended family. Perhaps they are cooking a festive dinner for two!

When someone has to attend a medical appointment, it is usually during working hours. Very few people are able to see their physician or attend a medical specialist appointment after hours.

Most workplaces have long adapted to this reality. Yet, therein lays another forgotten level of bias shown towards people without children. Two people in an office might have a medical appointment around the same time during the day. One of these people is taking their child to an appointment. The other, has no children and headed for an annual physical with the doctor.

A good manager will accommodate both parties, thereby keeping things fair. In many situations involving the employee with no children, you can bet they will be expected to reschedule that appointment in order for the manager to accommodate the parent first.

Many without children may also have a significantly harder time obtaining vacation and personal days from their employers. A few managers continue to work on assumptions that with no children, a person is somehow "less likely" to be sick.

Most politicians are also guilty of playing to the defined family dynamic. They view families as being people who have children. In election campaigns this becomes more obvious. Candidates will trumpet on how they want to work hard for your family, promising to make the world better for your children. I want my elected officials to start making improvements now. Why should I wait for a better world in the future when I am living in the here and now?

In the early part of the 2000's, Canada's Government introduced Compassionate Care Leave. This was seen as a remarkable step in a positive direction, addressing a growing senior population and the need to accommodate caring of loved ones by family members.

The idea behind "comp care leave" is to give citizens the opportunity to take time off in order to care for loved ones who are gravely ill. If you have so many hours of employment insurance time logged, you can qualify for up to six weeks of leave.

No employers in Canada are permitted to hold an employee back from applying for, and being granted time off for this purpose. In some work places where there is additional discretionary leave available, a person without kids may have more of a difficult time in getting that time off.

Many employers are still of the attitude that a person with no children somehow has all the time in the world with fewer responsibilities.

I am aware of stories where an individual without children would request an afternoon off to take an elder relative to a medical appointment, only to be told that since they don't have children, the appointment should have been made after hours.

The idea of the village being responsible for raising a child is a stale, outdated statement, reeking of dependency on constant social programming for all citizens. This is evident in the fact that governments in most democratic countries continue to offer more tax breaks for people who have children.

According to the Canadian Tax collection department known as the Canada Revenue Agency, the Canada Child Tax Benefit "CCTB" is supposedly designed to "help eligible families with the cost of raising children under 18 years of age".

Growing up, I was under the impression that in order to raise your family, you must go out and get a job in order to provide. Many view childcare allowance incentives paid as a way for people to make money off of having children.

Sadly, this has blown open a doorway where the wrong people are becoming parents for the sole purpose of financial gain.

Some parents who latched on to this culture of dependency will do everything to ensure they get by on parenting basics. This way they can never be criminally charged for failing to provide the necessities of life to the kids they have.

Canada also has the National Child Benefit Supplement, "NCBS", commonly known as the "Baby Bonus".

This horrendously nicknamed government handout implies it to be a reward for having children. This program is supposedly working in conjunction with the CCTB in determining how much money can be handed out to parents on a monthly basis.

In every single country where programs like these exist, you have special interest groups working within those countries that have spent significant amounts of resources in order to pollute the internet with complaints about how little money is handed out.

Many of these websites appear to give off different numbers when drawing comparisons amongst families with different income levels. Even some of the greatest mathematicians will probably find these numbers confusing! That being said, the Canadian government appears intent to keep these programs going regardless of who is in power.

How much enforcement and accountability is there ensuring this money is spent where it is supposed to be directed? Absolute Zero. Some parents will spend this money on their addictions and vices before they even think about using that cash to cover off childcare expenses. These monies are often treated as a monthly lottery win going straight to the wallets of parents.

Tax regimes in many countries reward those who have children while increasingly punishing those without them.

While it can easily be argued that those without children have larger disposable incomes, the tax benefits offered to parents will in some cases put more money into the hands of families with children.

Another fascinating prejudice often hurled at childfree people comes from those who base their reasons for having children solely on faith. Somehow it is supposed to be "a blessing from God" to have children.

With millions of different people making millions of different interpretations from religious scriptures, there are supposedly commands issued from the desks of higher powers that dictate having children is the sole reason we are here.

A common phrase I have heard from some people is that they will have as many children as "God will allow".

I remember someone who claimed to be a loving, kind Christian person who prided themselves on their ethics as being one of the people who took me to ask for going ahead with a vasectomy.

In the space of a few sentences and a short lapse of time, my soul was damned to an infernal imaginary furnace-like place where I would face punishment for what I did to my body. "God" did not want me to manipulate my body in such a fashion.

I was intrigued, how did these people have a direct connection to this "God"? Immediately I began to wonder how a person could become God's personal secretary and had such intimate knowledge of my private life. Maybe I am in the wrong business? I was preparing to ask for the phone number to his or her office but thought the better of it. Figured if I did get the number, I would end up speaking to a televangelist.

I ended the chat session politely, advising that if there was a God, he likely would not want me to bring children into the world. There is already enough of me here and no one else needs to be me.

Let us return to another social situation which is experienced by many but rarely expanded upon. I have heard of a few social conversations where a parent might be complaining about a myriad of issues related to their children.

These issues could range from having no intimacy time with their spouse; to being tired from night feedings and all of the running around they have to do. Everyone can agree that parents could tire easily from meeting the extra-curricular schedules. Most keep plugging away knowing that hopefully it benefits their children, especially if the kids actually want to attend these activities.

The childfree person in a conversation with a parent offers a polite and sincere "I understand" to the tired parent when the parent is talking about how exhausted they are. The parent, maybe irritated and worn from actually being tired, decides to ignite a flame by saying "You do not have children, so how can you understand?"

Here are a few facts this parent should have thought about before starting this verbal fight. People without kids have lives. They may have very busy lives. They too have groceries to buy, maybe pets that need to be fed and housework to be completed.

Maybe people without kids also have extra-curricular activities of their own to attend! Maybe they are artists who need to carve out time to devote to their crafts. Perhaps they have a glorious record of volunteer service work which they keep adding to.

The parent who foolishly elects to start the non-understanding debate is merely looking for friends to join them in a pity party. They know they are more likely to get this party since the majority of the world population intends to have children and create busy schedules for them. So a large group of sympathetic individuals is easily found.

Social Media has become the new breeding ground for some parents to cast out lines as they go fishing for pity parties. There are always more than enough willing friends and sympathizers happy to take the bait.

People who elect not to have children are often accused of being selfish individuals. Since when did caring for yourself and making your own decisions to make you happy become such a hateful thing? If being selfish is an act of self-care, I would say that having children could be one of the most selfish acts in the world.

Remember the parental unit in the previous chapter yanking out his wallet to show pictures of his future personal care attendants? He alluded to the fact he and his wife decided to have children in order to ensure someone would look after them in old age. That to me is being selfish no matter how you look at it.

In a world where there is not enough respect for the freedoms we take for granted, I believe that it is important to respect the choices of others.

Chapter 5
How Childhood
Experiences Influence
The Choice

Most people would probably be amazed and surprised at some of the reasons behind the choice to not have children. Some of the reasons could be a product of childhood experiences.

Some I have spoken to were willing to share vivid memories of abusive childhoods. There could be a natural fear that even though they survived the abusive childhoods, they do not want to become like their parents.

Many have also seen firsthand the damaging effects divorce can have on children. Kids are often used as pawns and are manipulated to take sides in matters during matrimonial deterioration.

Children often become the focal point of divorce proceedings and may be subjected to bitter and long legal wrangling. This is where kids may be forced to testify in court against one parent, possibly at the coaching of another. One cannot deny that in some circumstances kids put on the stand in a divorce hearing may end up revealing some truths that the judiciary may need to hear in determining a case outcome.

Even the youngest of the youngest can retain vivid memories of traumatic events. Many people I spoke to have told me they can easily play back parental fights verbatim as if they recorded them to tape.

Some who relive these moments will either learn valuable lessons by ensuring they will never put their children through the same thing.

Or, they may not have children altogether knowing they will never traumatize any kids with the kind of behaviours they witnessed growing up.

Everyone always has a fear of the inheritance of negative habits and behaviours their parents may have exercised. In our own quests for individuality, we may work very hard to formulate our own ways and learn from the bad habits of others. No one truly wants to inherit negative traits. Best thing to do is learn from them and go forward.

Bullying has been brought to the newspaper pages significantly in the last decade. Recognition of this epidemic problem also in turn may influence the decision made by someone choosing childfreedom.

A person may have been bullied throughout school, and like any other traumatic event remembers those moments clearly. Would they want a child of their own to possibly go through such horrendous terror and fear?

Parents who have to deal with their child being bullied have to deal with extra stress. They will worry more about their children while they are at school and hope they are safe from harm. Even with the raised awareness of bullying lies the potential threat that something could still happen.

With the digital age now also comes the threat of cyber-bullying. Kids have taken to Social Media in an effort to throw virtual mud at others. On the Social Media Sites, many kids are caught starting entire groups devoted to the hatred of individuals.

Just as alarming is the reality that supposedly mature adults are also using Social Media to sling mud in their divorce proceedings as they work through the legal system.

Have you ever heard of a parent trying to live through their own failed dreams through their children? I challenge you to attend or think back to any event where kids are the supposed stars.

You will see right away where hyper-parenting may very well be destroying the lives and interests of kids. Reality television has also given us a further glimpse into the lives of some of these people. Thanks to the wonder of television, we now see a dozen plus shows featuring parents who throw their children into constant cycles of beauty pageants and fashion shows, all in the name of living out failed dreams.

Parents also need to stop using their children for social gains. Once in a while, you might hear of parents who are telling their children to mix in with certain crowds solely for the benefit of the parents.

Too many parents are not giving their children a choice, especially when they are learning to empower themselves.

Let us refer back to competitive sports. There is one critical thing the parents at that hockey game I wrote about a few pages ago failed to consider. Free play teaches kids more lessons in sports than all-out competition. This takes much of the focus off of winning and back to the point of having fun. Parents forgetting this, have majorly serious issues beyond trying to live through their children.

I am a big believer that free play teaches kids much more in the way of learning teamwork and good sportsmanship. Organized sports and extra-curricular activities in general provide an excellent venue for kids to develop and further interests. I often wonder how many of the kids in these different things actually want to be there in these sports.

If parents asked these children what they would rather be doing, you probably would get many different answers from nearly all of the children asked. Children need to seek out their own interests, instead of being forced into things.

The kid at a piano recital, miserably walking up to the piano to play the same stupid song he had to practice over and over again is sitting there, unhappy.

He would rather grow his hair long and play louder styles of music. Or those hours of practice time could maybe have been spent outside playing sports with his friends.

The thought of fresh air and exercise! He hammers through this dreadful song, anxious to return to the solace of things he actually enjoys. When the song finishes, he gets up to walk back to his seat, passing his parents who have the plastered delusional hope on their face, indicating that they will push their kid into further study of music to live out their failed dreams of stardom. They dream of their young piano star becoming a Las Vegas headliner and giving them a comfortable living from it all.

Hyper-Parenting is defined as the overbearing presence of a parent in their kids' life. Some of this Hyper-Parenting carries over into very critical places. Overbearing Hyper-Parenting has cost children much sought after academic placements!

Parents will follow their kids to meetings with college and university recruiters. Some will view this as the parent being right in ensuring protection of their kids' interest. Others like me see this as a blatant interference in the decisions that should be made by the "child" who is now an adult.

Some of you will argue that if the parents are paying out of pocket they have a right to ask questions and have a say. Because of this, there is an increasing trend for kids to want to take on student loan debt by themselves to prove they can get through this chapter of life.

Hyper-Parenting is an exercise done by parents who have made children their lifelong projects. It is a mental activity fueled by the parents own failed dreams. Whether parents are costing their children academic placements or having phony dinner parties to set them up with the son or daughter of a rich doctor, these projects ultimately end up making the parent look like the fool to those who can spot it.

If a parent is still cutting up food for their child at the age of 10, they are taking steps to instill further fear into that child. Eventually the parent has to teach their child to use a knife.

Standing over them with their hands stretched out in the event they do slice their fingers open just is just anticipating the eventual inevitable. We all probably cut our fingers on a knife at some point when in the dining room or kitchen. An accident can happen!

These same children are instilled with significant other fears. The basic "don't talk to strangers" lesson could be drilled so far into the mindsets that a child may become afraid to talk to persons they are supposed to trust.

Parents often believe they are making decisions in the best interests of their children. Truth is many of these same parents are making decisions for their children that will serve the parents best.

They will ignore or completely forget the potential harm this level of interference will have. If the parent truly believes that they have raised the child well, then surely they will allow the now-grown child to make decisions on their own and even have them learn from any of the mistakes made.

This ultimately has become another deterrent for people not to have children. The childfree person may have been a victim of Hyper-Parenting and fear inheriting the same behavior as their parents.

They may also realize that they can still live out the life they want to lead and pursue their own goals and dreams, without the responsibility of parenthood.

Chapter 6
The Price

Bringing children into the world comes at a cost. The list of what those costs are seems to grow with the evolution of life. Childfree people are buoyed in their lifestyle decision by these cost implications.

There is an avalanche of information showing costs of raising children in Canada and the United States to be varying depending on the family income and living situation.

The costs are, not surprisingly, well into the hundreds of thousands of dollars. These numbers factor in everything from food and clothing, to paying for fees to keep children involved in interests, and in some instances paying for education tuition.

*In 2008, Statistics Canada listed total average expenditures for couples with children at $103,410.00 (for a single year). A one person household had an average of total expenditures at $37,904.00. If you double this amount to calculate a number for a two person household it would come out to be $75,808.00. By the math of the survey, this could represent the average expenditures for a childfree couple.

*Source – Spending Patterns in Canada, Statistics Canada Catalog #62-202-X

The over a hundred-thousand dollar per year expenditure is really quite astounding when you think about all the areas where this money would be spent.

So much goes into the cost of childcare, buying clothes, medical expenses, food, furniture and even home renovations that may be required to make room for new additions to the family. Consider clothing alone as a major expense. Children grow so fast that a significant amount of money is spent just keeping up with the wardrobe.

Parents involved in divorce situations where child support money is being paid are supposed to be accountable in proving to the court that the money is being spent for the childcare expenses.

Courts seem to think it's no problem attempting to enforce child support orders when the gavel hits the bench. However, most times accountability for where that money is spent is left wide open, with few rules and regulations actually in effect. Sometimes a person's word is considered well enough for a judge.

Regardless of what a person has to pay per month in child support, it is a cost. Sometimes the spouse receiving the child support payment is jobless or making too little to cover all expenses. In Canada, people paying child support are bound by Federal Guidelines and are required by law to pay a certain amount per month.

In cases among lower and middle income families, you might have the payer paying an amount of $225.00 per month per child. However it actually costs more to cover expenses for that one child.

Technically, the paying parents do not have to provide a single cent more to the receiver. I understand the frustration of many parents who strain themselves going into courts when they might legitimately need to seek more support dollars.

At the other end of this scale, you have the childfree person who might have more disposable income in their pockets. They will have significantly more breathing room in deciding and determining how they are going to allocate their expenses.

The choice to not have children brings about the accusation of being called "selfish". If you have more money at hand, you are able to better address your own personal needs more.

I believe firmly that selfishness should be positively defined as committing acts of self-care. Having more money to address your own needs and wants is an invigorating feeling. This is especially relevant when a person does not have to put a cent of that money towards childcare.

One of the most expensive costs of raising children can be the price of having children in daycare. To give you a more concrete idea of day care cost, let's use the example of private daycare at the cost of $35.00

per day, per child. Based on a five day week of care, this could add up to $9,100.00 per year.

To someone without children, this money might be a down payment on a new vehicle. It could also be the resources towards a temporary escape to a warmer client in the winter.

In the province of Quebec, they proudly trumpet a system of $7.00 per day daycare. In Canada, the idea that a taxpayer-funded National Child Care program should be in place versus the child care allowance still is a hot topic of debate. When the Quebec program started in 1997 it was at the cost of $5.00 per day. The mechanics of supply and demand worked their magic, with spaces filling up quickly and waiting lists ballooning. The rest of Canada and parts of the world have looked to Quebec as some sort of pristine example of affordable subsidized daycare.

Dual-income couples with young children in Quebec are actually farther ahead than a couple with the same scenario in Ontario. In 2005, a couple living in Gatineau, Quebec would have been at a significant advantage versus a couple living across the bridge in Ottawa, Ontario.

A working Quebec couple with three young children in daycare earning a combined living of $80,000.00 per year would have had a net amount of $48,628.00. By comparison, a couple across the water in Ottawa, Ontario would show a net income amount of $27,362.00. These numbers reflect the Gatineau couple having a 78% higher income thanks to Quebec's low-cost daycare and the significantly lower cost of housing.

The National Daycare Program for Canada spawned as an idea in the 1970's and has been dangled as an election platform carrot promised by successive governments and political parties since then. It has yet to see the light of day.

Those who made the promise and were elected to government woke up to reality, realizing that a Childcare allowance or bonus scheme would cost less and be more practical to maintain.

Many mothers and some fathers elect to stay home after their parental leave is completed in order to raise their children until they get to a certain age. This way, they can avoid the costs of daycare at the sacrifice of not bringing in extra work income.

Others will absorb their children into daycare for the purpose of helping them develop social skills. No one can deny that good quality daycare can be a very positive experience for children and parents alike. I sincerely hope that parents who have kids in daycare are getting their money's worth.

If the parent elects to return to work after parental leave, a significant part of their cheque will go to covering the daycare bill. You likely know someone, who is just going to work in order to pay for daycare.

Parents who are low income earners have to make the difficult decision whether to have one parent work or have one stay home. Many will return to work quickly if it means having a few extra dollars. There always seems to be sacrifices to make.

As a childfree person, I never saw myself as wanting to make that sacrifice, let alone many other ones. This is after considering the seemingly lifetime commitment involved in being a parent.

To a childfree person, subsidized daycare program ideas are part of a double-edged sword with very sharp ends. On one end they are being forced to pay tax dollars into a system to raise children that are not theirs. At the other end they are seeing tax dollars go into a system where cheques of a hundred bucks plus per month are freely handed out to parents to supposedly assist them with raising their children.

Meanwhile, someone without children cannot get as many tax breaks or as much assistance for things like furthering education. Government agencies always assume those without children have more money on hand for these kinds of things. It is respectfully, not always the case.

There is also the often forgotten demographic of unplanned pregnancies that are a result of criminal actions. The girls and women who are victims of these horrendous crimes may find themselves carrying more weight on the decision whether to keep or terminate the pregnancy. Protection and programs must always be made readily available to these victims. In some jurisdictions these programs are likely in need of more funding. I am more than happy to see tax dollars directed at keeping these kinds of support programs afloat. One cannot even begin to imagine the horrors that any victims of these crimes goes through.

There is also a relatively ignored danger lurking in the criminal justice systems of most democratic countries. This is a monster in the closet that cannot be defeated or even called out for battle.

There are women who are awaiting trial and disposition on criminal charges, suddenly becoming pregnant in hopes this will be used as a get out of jail free card. Men, who might also be working through the system when faced with jail, may use the new dad excuse to see if the judge may grant them some form of clemency.

The price in these scenarios expands to a much greater spectrum in the lead-up to and delivery of the courtroom's scene of sentencing. The justice system has to hope that another parent could be there for the child and perhaps the child could live without one parent for a while.

Do they want a woman to deliver her child in prison? Do they want to throw the mother of an infant behind bars potentially causing damage in the early stages of the relationship between mom and baby? Judges will ask themselves, will the child already be growing up in difficult circumstances anyway? Do they deprive someone genuinely remorseful for their actions of a relationship with their infant in the most important first few days of that child's life?

What about the cost to the public at large? Can a woman who kills an innocent person while drinking and driving can walk away from court to a sentence of house arrest or lengthy probation just so she can be there for her baby? Are the needs of the one outweighing the true value of complete public justice?

Parents who play the newborn infant card are hoping the justice system will spare them a deterrent sentence. How many of these cases are genuine? How many are open doors for offending parents to repeat criminal acts again after getting a slap on the wrist?

The cost to society is you have a parent who is spending time away from their children because of the choices they made. If the child does not have a suitable relative to go live with, then courts and agencies have to place these children in foster programs.

This adds further costs to the system. Then there is the worry about the child falling into the same patterns as the parent. Even if the parent manages to successfully be rehabilitated in the correctional facility, those that are involved in the child's life are on constant watch hoping that they stay away from run-ins with the police. This is how a vicious cycle can begin, and sadly continue, for so many.

Here is another classic and tired argument on the price of having children. Some people actually believe it is harder for a childfree person to meet someone they could spend the rest of their lives with.

How wrong they are! If anything, childfree people stand a much better opportunity of finding someone. Especially if they share the same desire to never have children!

Thanks to the a billion dollar per year industry of internet dating, people will proudly display their childfree badges in their profiles thereby attracting interest from other site users with similar lifestyle goals.

Here is another social scenario. You are out with a group of friends, and one of those friends is in a relationship that appears to be in significant trouble. At dinner, they spend the entire appetizer and main course rounds going through a litany of complaints about the things that are wrong with their spouse.

Once that list is complete and after everyone has had a chance to fill up their wine glass for the second time, that friend suddenly utters the show-stopper. "But that will all change once we have a baby".

The few people who remain interested in the conversation stop eating in perfect synchronicity. Then they look up to see which of their social circle is nodding in agreement at their friend.

The persons nodding in agreement have made themselves the target of an intervention come the next time they go to lunch as a group. The risk of friendship termination increases instantly.

As friends, the people surrounding that person are likely attempting to show compassion and care hoping to save the sanity of the person in trouble. They may be afraid to say anything for fear of losing that friendship, even though they may know they are working to try and prevent their friend from potentially making a major mistake.

This is diving into a shark pool known as band-aid births. People just automatically assume that bringing a child into the world will somehow change the entire dynamic of the whole relationship.

A relationship with serious problems will not magically improve by the entrance of a child into the lives of these troubled individuals.

If problems persisted for some time in that relationship, they potentially are going to persist for an even longer period of time. Birthing babies is often unfairly and pre-maturely considered a cure for problems in a relationship.

Band-Aid children may eventually become resented by their parents. I often wonder how resentful band-aid birth parents get when they know full well they had their children out of an attempt to salvage their own relationship.

Please do not think for a second I am placing the blame solely on the female gender for band-aid births. I believe that there is just as staggeringly a high number of men who thought having children would be the saving grace of a union.

These kinds of horrendous attitudes have been given full frontal display on platforms like television talk shows. I often wonder how many of these parents could sleep at night having such resentment for their children when they should be showing love and support that their children deserve.

Let us fast-forward to a few years later, same circle of people back at another dinner party. Band-aid baby is now about to start kindergarten. The complaining friend is preparing to divorce the spouse who was supposed to change once Junior was born. "I thought things would change once we had Junior but they didn't."

As everyone at the table completes their opening glass of wine, the friend continues quickly, covering any potential backlash. "I am so glad we had Junior though, and would not change that for anything even though we had so many problems and our lives were miserable."

If you have ever been in this situation, it almost feels like the person is saying they do not regret having children because they fear saying what is really on their mind.

Many people who do say they have no regrets having children are quick to say it out of fear of being thought of as a bad parent. I have no doubt that many parents who openly regret having children are wonderful parents and do everything they can to improve their mindset. Whatever it takes, they will do.

Sadly, many parents regret having these children because they were thinking their lives would get better. That kind of thinking just makes their attitudes worse and potentially causes problems for the children they are raising.

What if you are an only child and have decided children are not for you? Does your family situation mean the last name will stop at you?

The name and bloodline not carrying on can be a tough point of tension between family members. Some people may feel the immense pressure to have children on this basis alone. They feel they want to ensure the family name continues.

In some cultures, having large numbers in your family is some sort of a tradition. Therefore, the pressure to become a parent ends up being a paramount thing. This could be accompanied by a tremendous fear of disappointing the family. Especially if you have a solid relationship with them and you feel this could jeopardize family ties.

There are always consequences to the decisions people make in not having children. The potential negativity comes from pessimists who assume they are right in their thinking, absent research and facts.

Some family and friends may completely alienate those who choose not to have children.

Choosing to have children comes at a price, as does choosing not to have children. I have stated more reasons for not having them versus having them because I felt there was more of a case for me to be childfree. It is a personal decision, and people who make the choice deserve to have it respected.

Chapter 7

The Discipline Revolution & Evolution

How the times have seriously changed in the last several decades. I remember my Dad talking about how kids in his elementary school days would get "the strap" for doing something wrong.

That strap was a painful yet efficient deterrent to classroom craziness. Kids were generally afraid of the strap because it was known to cause significant pain. In the hands of a physically strong educator, that teacher instantly became a domineering force to be reckoned with. They become people looking to inflict pain in an effort to instill fear into children, and dole out a punishment accordingly.

Most families in Europe and North America no longer use corporal punishment as a method of disciplining their children. Use of the strap and caning gradually became frowned upon in these continents.

Precedent setting court cases of abuse in schools would forge the tone and direction of how corporal punishment would be viewed and administered. The perspective has evolved.

Using the strap or any physical form of punishment became criminal almost completely overnight. If a student is even tapped on the shoulder by a teacher today, the student may instantly look to form a criminal assault case. Educators now have to tread very carefully when enforcing rules.

Spanking, while still considered a form of corporal punishment, is still widely in use by some North American and European families.

More people now view spanking as a form of child abuse. Many parents still defend spanking as a necessary enforcement tool of household discipline.

Others have long denounced it, claiming it can cause significant trauma for children. A study reviewed on children subjected to spanking conducted by Duke University's Center for Child and Family Policy, concluded that spanking may have a serious negative effect on the mental development and behavior of young children.

Note: The Center has an extensive amount of reading material on many subjects. Much of this material will appeal to parents and non-parents alike. Read on at their website www.childandfamilypolicy.duke.edu .

This same study concluded that parents who spanked their children were often suffering from depression or significant stress. They may have been raised in conservative religious households where this form of discipline is more widely accepted.

In May of 2007, New Zealand's Parliament passed legislation that outlawed any form of corporal punishment on children. The country reignited the discussions on in July 2009 by holding a non-binding referendum. The ballot question is worded in such a way that I find quite humorous, so it's worthy of inclusion here.

"Should a smack as part of good parental correction be a criminal offence in New Zealand?"

87.6 % of voters in the country voted for the law to be overturned.

In Canada, the discussion of corporal punishment was renewed in 2002 with the Lucille Poulin case. "Sister" Poulin was a nun who ran a religious commune in central Prince

Edward Island.   She invoked religious reasons as the guiding force behind brutal beatings of children in the commune.

Poulin used a "rod" which was a wooden paddle, to hit the children under her watch repeatedly. Sometimes she would administer these beatings until the skin of the child cracked and bled.

At no time did she even consider the tremendous pain and suffering she was inflicting on these kids.   She maintained that her reasoning was religious-based and ultimately the punishment would prove beneficial to the children in her commune.

Poulin was unrepentant in her actions. The Supreme Court of Prince Edward Island sentenced her to eight months prison and three years of probation. Poulin was so adamant that she was doing the right thing that she gave a dramatic on the court record speech, proclaiming her love for God and the pride she had in knowing she carried out his "mandate".

The reality is that Poulin was a theocratic child abuser. She assumed through biblical interpretations that her actions were acceptable with no regard for the pain her actions caused.

Let's go back to talking about educators for a moment, for I believe they as well as child care workers have chosen some of the toughest work ever out of any occupation. They have to teach to a curriculum set by schools and are required to do everything they can within the program to ensure pupils get an education.

When they reach a point where they feel they have done all they can legally to enforce discipline in the classroom, they move on to get a vice principal or principal to see if they can step in to restore order.

If the discipline is still not effective from that point, the senior staffer of the school then calls home to where the discipline should have started all along. Those phone calls are essentially acting as a reminder to parents that they should be doing their jobs. The school then relies on the hope that the parent actually will enforce some kind of discipline on the child once they get home for the day.

I have heard from some educators that sadly the parents' response to such phone calls is, "What do you want me to do about it?" These are the same parents who will call the police when they give up on their children.

They will resign their position of being the household enforcers and expect police and judges to scare kids straight, in turn expecting courts of law to impose conditions, which then the parents are supposed to enforce. It is a twisted cycle.

Somewhere along the line, kids have to take responsibility for the choices they make and it is not always the fault of the parent. Kids can make bad choices based on the peer groups they might hang around, or other factors could play in. If the crowd of people is a negative bunch, then chances are the kid is more likely to attract trouble into their lives. This philosophy safely applies to adults as well.

Educators should not be given the task of handing down discipline to parents lacking the abilities to control their own children. Most parents agree that everyone has to adopt some sort of discipline strategy in order to effectively raise their children.

The general idea behind discipline is to correct children for mistakes they have made. Children need to make some mistakes in order to learn new things about life and how to cope with situations. This is part of the necessary development of life. Children are supposed to be encouraged with support, not disciplined by discouragement.

Disciplining a child is a ton of hard work. This is another critical and loudly championed reason for not wanting to have children.

I do not really want to play the bad guy in the home. I would rather be the reasonably cool uncle instead of a strict father. I rather treasure the idea of being an "Uncle Dann" who could get his nieces and nephews loaded up on caffeinated beverages, take them out to some fun places we all could enjoy and then drop them off to disgruntled family who will resent me for a twenty-four hour period, then quickly get over it because I gave them a break.

Instead, I would rather work with my dogs and cats.

When disciplining pets, owners want to work immediately to "correct" the animal for the negative action. Dog owners will work for hours on end training their dogs so they recognize a gentle pull is an act of correction. If the dogs are not wearing a leash, effective dog owners are also able to correct their dogs through verbal commands, which the dog can learn to recognize.

Cats tend to have a bit more independence. Correction for our feline friends might involve very simplistic deterrents such as the use of a light-pressure squirt gun full of water.

I often wonder if any parents have used squirt guns full of water on their children.

Parents using less forms of corporal punishment are moving towards more use of nanny-invented remedies like "time-outs".

I suppose the concept of a time-out is to take the child away from a few minutes of doing something they could be doing, like playing. Parents who have to enforce this rule are also required to warden watch their kids and ensure they actually stay in the designated time-out area.

Then as often demonstrated on television nightmare nanny shows, the parents come down to the kids level and offer some sort of reconciliation talk before the kid resumes their usual life living.

On these reality televised examples of discipline, the children will find themselves often back in the same time-out spot within minutes of having left it. Many parents who gave up on being strict enforcers will start negotiating with their children to get good behavior in return. Parents in these scenarios always appear to be giving up plenty in order to get their kids to provide them with a few minutes of peaceful bliss. This starts another cycle of enabling.

I have long observed grounding to be a complete joke and a waste of time. Watching parents take away something of their kids in order to send some message is in my view an ultimate failure. Telling a child they cannot have their stereo to listen to music is likely more of an incentive to send them out into the streets.

My parents knew that being able to play music was always a way to keep me off the streets.

From my own observations it seems that kids who are subjected to regular groundings are more likely to rebel in a much stronger fashion, in turn potentially getting involved in more trouble.

I recall a few horror stories of public humiliation suffered by parents who are forced to discipline their children on the spot in front of many people.

Instead of taking their children out of the public picture completely, they might start screaming at them in front of a crowd. Parents who pull this probably do not realize that they might be drawing more attention to themselves rather than the problems their children may have just created. They probably don't even think about the potential long-term affect that public humiliation will have on the kid.

Discipline is a trade that every single parent has to acquire. Sure, many do not even bother to learn the tools let alone the trade. Those that do are putting in several long hours learning what is most effective to them. It requires practice, patience and eventual perfection in order to make it work.

I would rather have too much time on my hands than be worried about offspring potentially stealing my car keys, sneaking out after dark, or climbing up any other mountain of trouble.

Chapter 8

Childfree & Childless

By this point you will have seen use of the term childfree dotted throughout this book.

Childfree are defined as people who have no children and exercise the freedom in choosing not to have children.

Childfreedom is a choice, involving weighing the consequences and saying no to bringing children into the world.

A previous but worn out term for childfree is childless by choice. Today the term childfree is the much more preferred and accepted moniker. Being childfree reflects the result of a lifestyle decision.

Having the word "less" next to child implies that something is lacking in that person's life. Choosing to not have children certainly does not make that person's life automatically lacking.

Someone who is childfree will readily submit that making that decision gives them a sense of personal enhancement. I look at my life as being more enriched because I have elected childfreedom. So, I have thereby chosen to enhance my abilities to do more things with my time rather than be a Dad.

There is a demographic of people who have no children and it is not by choice. Those who are childless by no choice are couples who are trying to conceive but for one reason or another and probably through no deliberate fault of their own, are unable to succeed at the conception process.

Most if not all of these reasons are medical in nature. These couples are referred to as being childless. I say this not to intentionally put them into a negative light, rather to shed insight into the fact that these are people who really want to and have tried to have children.

Sadly, their body science has barred them from becoming parents. They are lacking in the ability to produce and have children of their own.

It is easy to sympathize with the childless. They all want to become parents, maybe more so than the average couple. Most of the childless are really trying to have children, and come across as loving and caring people who want to start a family at any cost.

That is why we see many childless couples taking risks with costly and potentially unsafe fertility treatments. Even though many would argue the treatments have become safer over time, the element of risk is still very much there.

Medical science has advanced to a point where suddenly the childless may become expecting parents. Hopefully science will continue to evolve so the medical community

can continue to work on finding safe
fertility treatments. There is always
significant hope for those who
cannot conceive in the hard work
being put forth by researchers. I
hope that the right people get
access to these treatments, not the
opportunity seekers looking for half
hour spots on television.

Let's turn to adoption for a moment.
Adoption is a positive option for
those who cannot conceive.
Canada and the U.S. have an army
of adoption agencies that specialize
in adoptions from within local areas
to agencies with people on the
ground in poverty-stricken nations.

Many would-be parents are
increasingly adopting children from
third-world countries where poverty
and starvation run rampant. It is

admirable that instead of sending money through organizations that may provide minimal accountability for where funds are being directed, a handful of truly honest agencies and their people help to bring those children into a stable and loving environment. I believe firmly that all children, regardless of where they come from, deserve a shot at the good life.

The credibility of adoption agencies was recently called into question after two people behind Canadian-based Imagine Adoption were charged following an extensive police investigation.

Money that was supposed to be spent assisting parents in connecting with potential adoptions was instead directed to lavish vacations and home renovations. Families who were involved with this agency have thankfully had their cases taken over by another agency. However as of the time in writing this book, significant restitution is still owed to families whose resources were poured into Imagine Adoption.

Most of us feel for these families. I am fairly certain if statistics were calculated; many of these individuals are probably childless by no choice electing the "adoption option". I find it rather disheartening that many of these people probably borrowed and mortgaged themselves all in the name of trying to do something good for society.

I applaud the agencies and people who are working hard to make a difference in the lives of children. The victims of these scam agencies deserve justice, and deserve the opportunity to provide a child with a loving and caring home.

We should never consider gay, lesbian and transgendered couples as somehow automatically being childless. These couples who want to start a family are now less restrained thanks to a more educated and open-minded public in many countries.

A gradual decrease of global homophobia has resulted in many people now finally acknowledging that LGBT parents can provide just as loving of a home environment and family life for the children they either adopt or have through medically assisted procedures.

Over the course of the last decade, a handful of countries have acknowledged this and have started to relax adoption rules to put same-sex families on the same level as everyone else.

People tend to paint childfree and childless onto the same portrait canvass, identifying both sets of people as sharing the exact same viewpoints on having children. It is important that both definitions be defined clearly in order to distinguish the obvious differences.

A childfree person is more likely to be comfortable with the term "childfree" in any given social situation. In the case of someone who may be childless, it would be a significant difficult reality for the person to live with that term. You would be hard pressed to blatantly tell someone to their face that they are childless.

Childfree and childless may be better off identifiable just as people having no children. If a childless couple is fine with saying why they have no children then so be it. Everyone knows their own comfort levels. Childfree couples for the most part, are always ready to defend and explain their decisions.

Chapter 9

The Element of Regret

One of the most humorous things I have ever read on the subject of child-rearing was that the chances of people regretting parenthood were zero.

There are parents who have openly admitted to regretting that they brought children to birth. I believe firmly that there are a significantly large percentage of people who privately will admit it, but publicly will put on a positive show of face.

The concept of regretting having children is neither a new idea nor something that should be frowned upon when one expresses the admission. As difficult as it probably is to admit, I am willing to bet that many of the parents who admit this are probably good parents.

Perhaps knowing that they regret having children may have inspired them to make the most of the situation and do everything they can to be the best parents possible. The obvious reasons any parents would never want to admit an element of regret is the psychological damage this confession could cause to the children.

Could you imagine your parent admitting to you that they wish they never had children? No matter how wonderful a parent they might have been, it would be a horrible thing to hear.

On the other side of the regretful parent charts are the parents who wrongfully take this regret directly out on their children. They become bitter and angry towards their kids, blaming them for everything from interrupting life to shattering their dreams of self-aspiration.

Some parents also comment to friends and family wishing they had more information before they decided to have children. What I want to know is what information were they looking for? There is no real standard manual for how to be a parent.

There are dozens of parenting publications out there. Nine months of reading everything one can get their hands on will not prepare anyone for the world of parenthood. I guess it is certainly some sort of a start though. Parenthood to me sounds like it is a lifetime of learning. Often that learning is on the fly.

Another reason I chose not to have children is because I would likely be constantly worried about them. Parents will often talk frequently and freely about their parental worries. The over-anxious ones worry about everything from their kid's health and well being to schoolwork and their social lives.

One of the people who openly admitted regretting parenthood to me was talking about how she let the worry affect her life in such a negative way. Whenever her son was old enough to start going out and doing things with his friends, she would enter into a non-stop cycle of personal panic. I understood her reasoning and just concluded she probably was not the proper candidate for parenthood to begin with.

The over-anxious mother I just described is a classic example of the types of mental health problems one could develop possibly because of the choice she made. Her personality does not necessarily meet that of a parent who might be able to think and rationalize clearly. Chances are she probably had some sort of anxiety issues prior to having children.

Some parents wish they could get back the hours of sleep they lost dealing with child-related issues. This again, is a consideration in deciding whether or not to have children.

Anyone today can go online and find thousands of websites littered with stories of sleep-deprived parents. Sleep-deprivation can cause some serious health problems. I am willing to bet that there are a few parents who regret the hours of sleep they have lost. Many parents seem tired all the time. Sleeping in for a parent seems to be a luxury.

If a person has chosen to bring children into their lives and put aside their personal dreams and goals, most learn to live with the choice.

Most people who have children have made tremendous sacrifices. But I am not of the view that a person's entire life should somehow be put on hold just because they become a parent. Parents will use their children as an excuse for stopping themselves from going further in life. They should be able to continually pursue their dreams and passions just like everyone else.

If there is an additional mouth to feed, then the parent has elected to own the responsibility of feeding that mouth and raising the child attached to it properly. No one should ever feel the need to regret having children. More parents need to take personal action to make their own lives enriching and rewarding outside and inside the roles of parenthood.

If the parent truly has the drive to do what they really want in life, they should find a way to make it happen while balancing their parental responsibilities. The children will then learn by example this is a very positive way to live.

I no longer care to hear negative attitude mothers who say "I wanted to become a doctor but once I had the baby I decided to become a mom instead". Whenever you hear this story, most of the time it sounds like the parent is just settling for the scenario. Instead of settling and regretting the decision later, parents should want to and continue to follow whatever paths they somehow think were thrown out the window.

I believe being childfree is a decision that is pretty much firm, once made. People like me who have gone the extra mile to ensure sterility have taken out an insurance policy on the choice.

Even when some people proceed that extra mile, I realize it will never completely eliminate the possibility of regret later in life. I acknowledge fully that there is a very slim chance I may regret not having children, someday.

In the same ignorant conversations I have with people who somehow know for sure I am going to regret it later, they then start to invoke their own medical knowledge of the vasectomy procedure. Saying things like, "It is not 100% effective."

Well I had to hand it to them there! For a few brief seconds I want to give them their moment in the sun. The last word however goes to me. "You are right." 'It is not 100% effective, it is 99.8% effective!"

Believe me; I am more than happy to take that 0.2% chance. I count that small percentage as the same likelihood of me ever changing my mind. If all of a sudden I am going to become a father I will still have been happy to have taken that gamble.

Top 5 Reasons I am told I will regret not having children

1. *You will have no one to take care of you when you are older.*

2. *You will have no one to carry on your legacy.*

3. *You will miss out on the "joys" of parenthood.*

4. *You will be lonely when you are older.*

5. *You will deprive others in your family of nieces, nephews, cousins or grandchildren.*

When it comes to having a legacy, why would I want someone to carry on a legacy if I create one? Sure it would be nice to inspire others to take their lives in a positive direction, or support causes I am proud to back.

But I would want people to do those things as individuals. People should want to blaze their own trails. I never seek to pick up where someone in my family has left off. I seek to do things and live life my own way.

My support for animal rescue causes was inspired partly by my Grandmother. Am I carrying on her legacy in giving so much to these causes? No. I am taking inspiration from her and building based on that inspiration.

So I am promoting care to animals as an individual, making my own legacy and being happy with what I can contribute to the cause. If others want to follow my example, it should be with the recognition that they are doing it as themselves.

Looking at reason 3, it is the alleged "joys" of parenthood work that act as one of the deterrents to having children. Parenthood by definition is a major life commitment involving significant sacrifices one must make. I am not in any way comfortable putting my aspirations on hold in order to raise children.

There are parents who are able to balance raising their children in pursuit of their goals. To those parents I would tip my hat and say congratulations on being able to accomplish what many parents have walked away from.

People who chose to take a pass on having children are doing so in order to enrich their own personal joys. For me, the number of any supposed joys of being a parent would pale in comparison to the number of joys and possibilities I could experience as someone without kids.

The idea that having children will automatically ensure elimination of elderly loneliness is laughable. Especially to those who are able to take significant pleasure in those peaceful moments of "you" time. Some people love to have their lives completely to themselves, while others may want constant socialization and company.

My want to travel to different parts of the earth, keeping up on the lives of family, friends and colleagues, desire to read as many books on topics of interest as possible, and the drive to be a working writer for the rest of my life will be more than enough to prevent any loneliness from setting in. My status as a pet-owner "Animal Dad" will be permanent as well.

Finally, another reason to have children should not involve providing elders in your family with younger bloodline objects to be proud of. If you hear of anyone who is obsessively pressuring their children to give them grandchildren, then they could be creating a potentially divisive situation. Pressures from within the family (within social circles for that matter) for production of children could ultimately turn people away from each other. The want to have children should be from the parents themselves and no one else.

A person should not have children just to breed them into available vacancies in the family.

The element of potential regret is present in all aspects of every choice. It exists as a bit of a nag that might try to throw you in an overwhelmingly different direction than the one you are travelling.

Truth is, most that go about choosing not to have children have genuinely researched the choice thoroughly. Even though I chose childfreedom at an early age, I still went ahead and did some significant reading on the what-ifs and potential regrets.

The potential regret factor for me is as mathematically close to zero as possible. This is because my examination of the possible regrets has been enlightening and educational. I have worked hard to ensure there will be no regret at all. Hopefully, I will be right.

Chapter 10

Directions

As someone who has decided not to have children, I share some of the same opinions that many others without children have. There are viewpoints that someone without children may want to share, but are afraid to out of the fear of being dismissed from social circles. It is time to share some of those collective thoughts and suggested directions.

Childfree people, empty nesters and those who are childless, deserve some sort of tax relief equal to breaks that parents get. The handing out of a baby-bonus and childcare allowance is seen by many as a token reward for having children.

In some cultures, having kids is the only way to ensure old age security. India for instance, has no Social Security Program. Many women end up looking after their in-laws. Because of the large population of men India is now paying for parents to have daughters. This is said to ensure that more women are available to look after the aging population. I find it rather disheartening that there are still cultures all over the world that delegate women to caregiver homemaker roles and nothing else, especially when they deserve equal treatment.

There is no clear evidence that any birth incentive programs, whether it be the program I just mentioned from India, or the made in North America schemes, are actually working.

There is no accountability in the North American Programs I referred to. The governments that run them are blindly assuming this money is all actually spent on necessities related to the raising of children.

Accountability seems only to be considered when divorced parents go through the court systems which arrange for (and orders) child support payments. Even then, there is no complete aoccountability on where and how money is spent.

Courts have a difficult time already collecting from so called "deadbeat" parents.

Judges and social program administrators should impose stricter accountability action on parents who are in receipt of child support money proving what that money goes towards. Even a grocery store receipt showing a quart of milk should become part of that paperwork.

A few of you will read this and argue that the courts are bogged down with "frivolous" things and would not have time for things like this. This idea is a long-overdue and far from a joke treatment.

These ideas are not frivolous if they are in the best interest of the kids and for transparency in custodial arrangements. If a parent is not paying child support, they need to pay up. If the parent receiving support payments is not spending the funds properly, they need to be held accountable to the courts for any misuse.

Speaking of courts, let us look at doing something about domestic violence matters and how they could have an additional element of consequence attached to those committing violent acts.

In Canada, when the police are called to a domestic violence situation with children present, police will send a form to the local child services agency. This puts child protection officials on notice and allows the agency to open a file on the family. Documents are then generated for a file which may show that kids are being subjected to treatment in a negative home atmosphere.

In addition to this procedure, we should go a step further. Respective governments should introduce and pass laws that would allow the offending parents to be charged for subjecting their children to these situations.

These situations essentially could be classified as emotional abuse. Children who are subjected to this kind of atmosphere can develop both short and long-term problems. Most disturbing is that exposure to these environments can have a major effect on how they develop in their own personal relationships, even carrying these behaviors and attitudes through school and into the workforce.

It is horrendous enough that a parent in a domestic violence situation is criminally charged with doing something unthinkable such as pushing, or striking the other parent of their children, someone they are supposed to love.

It is just as bad that a child can be subjected to witnessing these horrors. If police arrive on a situation and are unable to lay a charge against the parent for physical violence, with strong evidence they should be able to proceed on doing something against one or both parents just for what they have subjected their children to. Verbal violence is still violence. If one parent was making efforts to shield the kids from harm that evidence would hopefully turn up through the course of an investigation.

Let's look at an example as to how those without children can exercise their voice to an opinion on municipal election days.

In Canada, most municipal elections coincide with elections of school officials.

In many places in the province of Ontario, you have the option of voting for school board officials from three choices. Firstly, you have a regular public school board, which represents the majority of educational institutions in the area where most kids go to school.

Secondly, many places will have a local Catholic school board. This organization represents faith-based English language speaking schools that have a combined mandate from parents, the Ontario Ministry of Education and the Catholic Church.

Finally, a person can vote for someone to the board of the Francophone separate school board. This is the body of administrators that assist to run French immersion schools.

When I was living in Ontario, by default and no direction, our portions of property tax dollars were sent to the local public school board. Come election time, my wife and I have promptly not marked an X beside the names of anyone running for the public school board. Even if a friend or a family member was running for one of these school boards as a trustee, I would refuse to put down a mark.

This is one way we speak up and out against the fact that we have no direct say as to where our money will go. In March of 2011 as part of book research, I submitted to the City of Thunder Bay a request that our portion perhaps go to the municipally run SPCA animal shelter.

Those without children should not be responsible for paying for the education of children they do not have. By that same token, empty nesters have paid their share and should have the option of directing those monies to another municipal department.

When I queried the local municipality in Thunder Bay as to the reasons why we are required to pay this money, the answer I received was not one of surprise.

The official elected to merely point me in the direction of reading Ontario's Education Act. This kind of an answer is a "because the government says so" type of response. So the answer I was left with is because the government says so, it is what it is.

It seems no one can ever question the reasons why portions of property taxes are directed towards schools. Rather we are just expected to do it blindly and not question it because we live in a society dependent on natalist philosophies.

A read of the aforementioned Act, a stale and dusty piece of legislation last updated in 1990, it seems completely muddled and unclear as the day it was drafted. One would probably have to bring it to a lawyer to have it interpreted for them. I suspect even some of the brightest legal minds in the country would even have trouble with how the Act is worded.

When I contacted Ontario's Ministry of Education to query them about the wording of the Act, and ask their opinion as to why this scheme favours parents and strong-arms those with grown or no children into paying where they should not have to, the answer I received was something I expected. The following response was merely a re-stating of a decrepit point of view. This is taken verbatim from their reply to me.

It is important to recognize that all of society benefits directly or indirectly from a high-quality public education system. For this reason, taxpayers in Ontario contribute to the funding of public education through education property taxes. It is also important to recognize that today's students are tomorrow's taxpayers who, through the course of their working lives, will be supporting a variety of government programs and services that are available to all Ontarians.

Someone was paid a lot of money to write that response. The age-old argument favouring this tax structure which governments and most people will give reverts back to the village raising the child. Childfree, childless (and empty nesters for that matter) are bound in law to pay property taxes to their municipality towards a local school to pay for the education of children they do not have.

People who are paying rent are still essentially paying property taxes through to fund education services as well. Most landlords pass on the costs of paying for property taxes onward to tenants.

A supplementary argument is also that we should be paying for the future scientists and doctors who very well could be responsible for one day prolonging our lives.

No. If the child has an interest in going into these professions, it should and must be encouraged.

Yet the principle of responsibility is worth a reminder. The parents are responsible for encouragement of that interest and possibly for furthering the education of those children.

Part of that encouragement must include funding of that education or assisting them in obtaining student loans in order to finance the higher learning.

Let me state right out that I do understand completely the necessity of student loans. I was one of many who had to obtain student loans. Part of the reason I did so was out of the want of responsibility to be able to pay those loans back and say "I did it".

These student assistance programs are very necessary, and I know full well that many parents, despite their best intentions, cannot afford to fund higher learning for their children.

During my time working at an order desk for a wholesale supplier in Calgary Alberta, I met an older tile installer who always seemed to be working. Rory worked six solid days a week. In a busy housing market where homes were being built and renovated at rapid paces, you could see where this guy would be getting a ton of work.

Somewhere towards the end of my tenure in this job I remember asking him why he worked so much. It seemed like he never could take a day off. He replied that he was so used to working that he just kept on going, even after putting all eight of his children through college.

I am always astounded at the thought of someone putting one child through life and learning. But eight surely is something to be even more astounded by. My jaw still on the floor, I took to asking him why they just did not get student loans. I unfairly assumed that with eight children he might be inclined to push them towards obtaining funding on their own.

Rory had immigrated to Canada from the Caribbean with his entire family. He said he always managed his money well and knew that he would be able to afford higher learning for his children. So he never felt it necessary to push his kids towards obtaining student loans. So a little extra work, and he felt he could assist all eight of them.

In 2001, then-Premier of Ontario Mike Harris announced and subsequently implemented a private school tax credit for parents who were sending their children to private institutions.

This tax credit allowed for parents to receive money for sending their kids to a private school. The credit was to max out in its' fifth year to $3,500.00. This was reflective of half the actual cost of keeping a student in the publicly funded educational system at the time.

The Ontario private school tax credit was meant to give some sort of credit to parents who were paying for the private school tuition, but also give them a tax break for what they would have contributed in tax dollars to the public system.

The children who are placed in private schools create spaces in already-strained public systems. While this tax credit was quickly cancelled in 2004 with the election of a new government, the idea is still given much discussion as a historical examination of progressive policy.

The reason I mention this tax credit is to draw attention to the idea that a tax credit to those with no children and empty nesters appears not really to be as far out of reach as some might believe.

Unfortunately, adaptation of a tax break like this is still not a popular idea.   Instead, the overwhelming majority of the population expects the village and the government to be the proverbial Nanny from cradle to grave.   This means everyone is expected to take part in raising children no matter where the originating DNA is spawned from.

If those without children were permitted to have their share of property tax dollars go perhaps to municipally run animal shelters, few of those shelters would have to aggressively solicit donations.

Responsibility of raising a child lies with the parents.   Most parents accept that responsibility willingly. They make mistakes, learn from them and try to be better. It can be argued that a large percentage of parents do not accept those responsibilities.

There could be a million reasons as to why some parents are utter failures at their jobs. Even so, if one makes the decision to bring children into the world, they should accept full responsibility.

We live in a glorious age of being able to benefit from the wisdom of a substantial senior population. Yet instead of accommodating them with things like more parking spaces, many spaces are now reserved for expecting mothers and or families with young children.

I can recall many busy holiday shopping seasons where I watched in anger while seniors would drive around a parking lot waiting for one of the two accessible parking spaces in a row to open up. Meanwhile the four per row expectant parent parking spaces are full.

I would sometimes watch as people would park in these spaces while the senior cars would proceed to the next row looking for the open space in resigned frustration. Then in those same moments, I would start to see someone struggling to make their way up to the entrance of the supermarket store or mall entrance. Many of them would be walking with assistance from a family member or with the aid of a walker device.

Surely the dignity of our seniors is perhaps worth a hell of a lot more than parking spaces for expectant parents. Despite the physical limitations pregnant women can endure during pregnancy, being pregnant is not considered a disability by physicians. If an expecting mother is experiencing complications that limit her walking, she can obtain a temporary permit in order to use an accessible space.

According to a never-ending array of baby and pregnancy-related websites, many of which contain contributions from doctors, midwives, doulas and others involved in the care of expecting mothers, light walking is something that can and apparently should be done throughout the entire pregnancy. Light walking of a few extra steps in a parking lot apparently benefits both mother and child.

I would prefer to see those pregnancy spaces be converted to accessible parking spaces. Surely we can and should accommodate our growing senior population and also provide enough accessible spaces for those who require use of devices such as a wheelchair or walker.

During a time when I watched more television, I made a point to watch some of the parents who had the brilliant idea of taking their problems to talk shows.

Observing how some of these people acted and hearing about how they go about parenting would often prompt the thought that parents should have a license.

During a time when I was recovering from car accident injuries, watching Maury Povich's talk show would become the best possible example for my idea of parental licensing. Seeing these parents come onto a national platform and tell their personal stories of tragedy and DNA uncertainty would give me tremendous amounts of laughter.

All that kept going through my mind was how could these parents put the children they supposedly love through this kind of nonsense?

In the real world before us all, the same question could be asked of parents who put their children through hell every day for other reasons. There never seems to be shortages of stories about children who are abused yet still remain in the homes of the abusers. One can appreciate that in many cases the kids may not be able to speak or no one around them is picking up on signs of danger.

When kids are taken from the home by child protection agencies, many of those children are released back to their parents a short time later. Often this is with minimal court intervention or any suggestions of where the parents could improve themselves. Many people who might hear these stories will shake their heads and suggest that parents should be licensed before they could even have kids.

What a great thought this is! A parent that has to attend mandatory training in their chosen role! Having to sit through a classroom of government regulated parenting seminars written by doctors and child health specialists.

Let us go referencing back to the Canadian system of the childcare allowance and bonuses versus a National Day Care Program. A National Day Care Program would be a government run system made fully accountable to a Federal Ministry overseeing how it operates and setting high standards for how providers are to run services.

If we are to keep allowing governments to issue these hand-outs to parents, how about ensuring mandatory parenting programs through local health authorities are made available?

If the parents pass the program then they can qualify for any allowances. I can hear some of you already asking how this would be paid for. My response would be since the government so readily hands out money on birthing incentives, they can cover parenting programs and even licensing using existing revenue.

Many single-issue agenda social groups surrounding parents and children are always calling for things to be changed so more money and programs could be provided for parents to raise their children. This is fine by me, as long as you are not taking that money from my pocket. Do not punish me for my lifestyle decision and expect me to contribute to the raising of your children.

The idea of a stand-alone National Day Care Program could be made efficient and would be an alternative to paying out these rewards for having children. In addition, those funds should come from parent generated tax revenues. If the baby bonuses and child care allowances are to be kept flowing into the pockets of parents, then subsidized daycare should be eliminated.

If there is to be a federally funded day care program minus child care allowances, then only parents should be paying for that program.

Let's take all the childcare allowance and give it directly to the providers. The governments have said the point of these programs is to assist parents in the raising of their children. Parents in the lower-income brackets who are having trouble making ends meet would see childcare allowances put towards needed daycare services, and the money for funding those services could be contributed through dollars collected from families with children. Those who have no children should never have to pay for the education of children they do not have. Further, empty nesters should stop paying education taxes once their children are either out of public school or they turn whatever the country determines is the "of age" number.

Someone suggested to me that if only parents are left to raise children minus participation from the village, could this lead to a less-educated society? I would say no without any hesitation. If more parents took on an active role in their kids' education, I believe we would see a dramatically positive turnaround in the way school programs are delivered.

I like to believe that most parents have the best intentions in mind for their children, even though we know some are far from that mentality. Parents who raise children well may inspire their kids to pursue further education, chasing the life well worth living, doing what they really want to do and be good contributors to society.

Every once in a while, I delight in reading stories about children who overcame having delinquent parents and have gone on to bigger and better things. Surely there are hundreds upon thousands of tales like these that go unwritten and unnoticed.

I understand that the idea behind referencing the village raising the children means others around the community having indirect input into the direction children might take.

In every community, the village will have a group of persons who perhaps some children may really look up to for positive reasons. Maybe that local sports hero, or the great neighbour who brings the most delicately prepared sweets to community bake sales is someone who by nature, inspires well being in local children.

This is all well and good, but does not mean that they are raising those children. Chances are they may be raising children of their own and living life. They and others like this must really just be choosing positive pursuit usually in their own interests, minus the intention of being a figure of community guardianship.

One of the greatest benefits that come with parenthood is maternity leave. In Canada this benefit was recently extended to fathers thereby changing the name of the program to parental leave. That first year proves to be so important in a child's development. Now parents have the potential to both be home during this critical stage.

I believe that this is a commendable advancement as society does more to recognize the equal importance two parents must play in raising their children.

So why not offer some programs to those without children? Those who have chosen not to have children should be given some more incentive where they could take time off to further their studies without having to re-mortgage their lives. If parents are given ample opportunity to make the lives of their children better, those without children should be given similar treatment and assistance in order to enrich and advance their own paths.

Any parent in Canada who applies for post-secondary studies financial assistance is able to obtain additional funding above and beyond any childcare allowance along with baby bonuses to cover provider care costs.

Many of the people I went to post-secondary studies with were able to cover off their childcare costs without having to take a part-time job to supplement living expenses.

Meanwhile, I went to a full days worth of classes, left school to work a part-time job until 9 p.m. many nights, and it still was not always enough to cover everything.

The student finance assistance system just assumes that people with no children should somehow be able to afford extra towards their education.

It seems that a person who has children is more than likely to receive more assistance to attend post-secondary studies. Some parents who might have a better financial backing could still get more student assistance from their respective government programs than the average person without kids.

I briefly touched on the idea of parental licensing a few paragraphs back, so let's explore this further in depth. You need a license to own a dog, but any person can have children without meeting any set prerequisites.

The idea of mandatory licensing for parents is a glorious dream but seems like an impossible policy to implement. The idea of parental licensing is fairly straight-ahead and sensible. You need to hold a piece of laminated paper or plastic and meet the requirements of holding that card in order to drive a car, operate certain types of heavy machinery and be in certain professions where you are expected to have a significant modicum of knowledge. So why not have a license to be a parent in order to protect your children from potentially dangerous neglect?

Most of the reasons this kind of set-up will not work are attributable to cost. The relationship between individual and government would also see a major irreparable fracture among the majority population.

People feel that they automatically have sort of controlling right over their children. So this concept could be viewed as an intrusion onto that person's rights and freedoms. If licensing were to exist, government would only need to intervene on the parents if there was some legitimate necessity to do so.

So child services agencies could become even more of an enforcement branch than ever before. In the current day and age, many child service groups are quite terrified to intervene in situations. Because of the ever-changing adaptations of law, many child protection workers tread very carefully in order to minimize liability.

The whole idea of licensing would not be to have a government agency teach people how to be parents. Rather, it would exist in order to prevent parents from inflicting negligence on their children. The probability that a licensing body could even come to a mutual agreement on what would be defined as good parenting is minimal to zero.

This whole question could be a separate lasting argument all by itself. People have different definitions of what is defined as good parenting. Sometimes those values are interpreted and based on faith, family traditions or supposed standards in "classic" parenting literature.

I suspect anyone reading these pages who are subjected to regular horror stories of poor parenting may agree with the licensing idea.

American Philosophy Professor Hugh Lafollette published a more comprehensive and complete analysis of the parental licensing idea in the winter 1980 edition of

*"Philosophy and Public Affairs".
This is a brilliantly written piece
which best explains both sides of
this idea.*

*A copy of this piece can be viewed
on Professor Lafollette's website at
http://www.hughlafollette.com*

*I acknowledge Professor Lafollette's
work for his research and writing on
this sub-topic, and thank him for his
insight during the writing of this
book.*

I appreciate that many of these
ideas for change are nearly
impossible to implement from a legal
and cost perspective. The natalist
society automatically wants to look
at encouraging those who have
children, while discriminating (albeit

sometimes unknowingly) against those who do not.

There is a growing frustration among the childfree community at the lack of acceptance and understanding of this choice. Childfree people have lives, families, and interests. Meanwhile most empty nesters have done their part on the parental stage and are now pursuing life as parents of grown children.

Hopefully they have done their jobs well and have raised children to head out on their own ready for life. Empty nesters are now able to focus on a usually quieter and less hectic life while maintaining interest in the lives of their children and perhaps grandchildren.

That is, if their kids make the decision to have their own children....

Chapter 11

The Summary of Summaries

People without children have lives. The workplace needs to think equal in consideration of policies they exercise towards employees so everyone is on a level field in the workplace.

Most companies are often unaware that they are automatically being more accommodating to those with children. There is an auto-assumption that someone without children should rarely miss work as they have perceived fewer personal commitments.

Just assuming that someone without children is perhaps always going to be available for an emergency work situation and overtime is narrow-minded. The so called "family friendly" companies are merely identifying themselves this way to alleviate any possibility of offending employees with children.

Little to no consideration of those without children in the corporate commandeering of decisions still runs rampant. Parents are still given preferential treatment when every person is supposed to enjoy an equal level of treatment by superiors and colleagues.

With increased awareness of racism, bigotry and equality issues came the developmental need for sensitivity training. Sensitivity training is supposed to make us more aware of personal bias and proposes solutions on how to rid one of biased perceptions. Originating in the late 1940's, sensitivity training has become a business worth several million dollars a year to human resource consultancy practices.

Sensitivity training is actually mandated in many workplaces. The training appears to have been put in place to respond to growing concerns about equality in the work place. The idea behind this kind of training is to make companies and organizations appear to be showing signs of respect towards all people. This is whether they succeed in the training goal or not. It is still there to at least cosmetically make it appear that something is being done.

This is especially evident in the public sector, where strict policies on respect and equality are preached by highly paid consultants over a one day training session in a fancy conference room. The intention of this kind of training is definitely honourable and ultimately has become necessary to address deep and often divisive issues.

Where almost every single workplace fails is the lack of consideration given to anyone who has no children as part of this training. There is still an alarming level of bias against those who have no children. It is another venomous form of intolerance that should be remedied with antidotes of education and acceptance. *Families without children are still a family.*

Another common misconception is that all those who are childfree somehow do not like kids. We can all agree that some people do not like children. Just because a person chooses to not have children does not mean they would dismiss them if they entered their field of vision.

To elaborate further, many people who do not like children are not specifically targeting every child as part of a group. They may just feel uncomfortable being around them in some situations.

I would say to each of you that after a while children are supposed to know and understand respect for other humans (and animals) they share the earth with. There are points some parents get to, when they decide to give up completely (but would never admit to parental resignation) and suddenly the government becomes the parent to those children through many programs that are offered.

Finally, some people who crave peace and quiet may be uncomfortable around children because they know that eventually, children will scream and children will cry.

I do not see how this can ever be something personal against children. What I do see though is the idea that someone may really crave silent stability and will do anything to safe guard it. If things get too hectic, that person can just leave the room and go somewhere quiet. These are the kinds of children people may feel uncomfortable being around. It is rarely, if ever, personal.

Anyone who has chosen against reproduction should not be sequestered outside of the societal circle. The level of intolerance against those without children still appears to be high due to a lack of understanding.

When I referred to the impossible changes and future directions in previous pages, this states a reflection of the difficulty in achieving those changes. Over time, I very much believe that positive changes in favour of those choosing not to have children can happen.

Most people who question the decisions of childfree do not give consideration to what they have said in those situations. They just assume that their comments and opinions are the right ones. Since many people may say the same things and show the same level of bias, they feel there are little to no consequences from the blatantly intolerant remarks some people will say.

Saying an enthusiastic "no" to having children is a major proclamation. Making this decision for some may not be easy. Others may have made the choice in lightning quick time.

For greater understanding of Planned UnParenthood and the choice of no children, ignorance must be replaced with acceptance, and intolerance with understanding.

Afterwords and Acknowledgements

June 2015

Most authors when they decide to re-write portions of a book might wait longer than three years to do it. Much has changed since September of 2012 when I first released this book. The idea of revisiting the script was far from my mind. It all changed one evening.

I was reading a wonderfully detailed critique from a reader while looking over some ideas for newer content. It dawned on me that with all of the additional experience gained over the last few years, maybe it was time to really look at this book one more time. To give it another read through. To see how far I have come as a writer who has now significantly more experience. As you will see below, the original idea was formulated at the end of 2009. So the writing really started right then, making the content older than the nearly three years since first published.

The overall content has seen few changes. Some of the language and formatting was cleaned up and I removed as much of the self-deprecating humour as possible. I've grown rather tired of beating myself up and see full on how it can come back to haunt me. It's good to laugh at yourself, but not all the time.

The number of resources devoted to childfree and childless related issues is growing. One of my personal favourites is nonparents.com where I have enjoyed the privilege of contributing to the growing amount of insightful content. Everyone should check out the site and see how many of the articles you can relate to. The site encourages people to submit their own stories and provides ample opportunity for reader comment and discussion.

The response to this book has been and continues to be, incredible. The feedback I have received from readers is overwhelmingly positive. One of the great accomplishments for me over the last few years was to win International Childfree Man of The Year in 2014. This book certainly played a role in my winning the award. It is an award recognizing contributions of people who have promoted issues surrounding the choice not to have children. I would point out that myself and other award winners also promote and discuss matters surrounding pro-choice and those who cannot have children.

Thank you to everyone, and I do mean everyone for your support. Thank you for buying and thank you for reading. For me to name everyone on these pages without forgetting a few would just be impossible and I would not want to leave anyone out.

Below is the original afterword as written in 2012. I felt it best to leave it in as it best captures the sense of accomplishment and gratitude that I felt when the book was first completed.

Dann Alexander
June 10, 2015

Original Afterword - 2012

Boxing Day 2009 was a happily hectic gathering of family at my in-laws' home.

Several family members were over with children in tow. Instead of throwing myself into the fray of children running everywhere, I elected to keep a chair occupied in the heated garage and inhale an appalling amount of second-hand smoke. It seemed like a small price to pay to have much needed peace and quiet. (*Note – Even a busy household of children is no excuse for putting your health at risk. I have put this note in during final edits of the book as a polite disclaimer)*

One of the gifts we received that December was one of those one-cup coffee makers. Even though I prefer tea, this machine's ability to make good quality java gave me great incentive to keep pouring cup after cup. With any generous amounts of caffeine comes the certainty that one will get insanely hyperactive, and for a long period of time.

Somewhere after I lost track of how many cups I had drank my thoughts were wandering. I remember thinking about the crazy busy life of a parent and how I carry a sense of pride that I chose not to have children. Maybe the caffeine was taking me on some exploratory journey, helping me to look for a book idea worthy of writing.

The smoke-filled garage fell silent in my mind. My ability to tune out everything around me was stronger than ever as the idea for this book clicked. A book about the choice of not having children would be a natural fit and something I figured many people would read.

Since my coffee cup was empty, I took a moment to run through the middle of the foray into the kitchen where my wife and a refill of coffee would be. Quietly I told her of the idea for this book. Her reply was one of agreement. She didn't expect me to come in with a writing idea. I was sure she was expecting me to ask that we go home, given the chaos.

I spent the rest of that evening thinking about what I wanted this book to say. It developed into more of an all-around look at those without children whether they chose it or not.

A few days later, I started to fill notebooks with ideas and a draft outline.

There are many printed publications about the choice to have or not have children. In addition, readers can do a significant amount of research online through various support groups. I decided not to read any of the books already on the market before writing this book. I want to respect the authors who already have their product out there and give readers something very fresh from a singular perspective.

The ultimate goal of this book has been to be a vehicle for education and entertainment. This is my take as a person without children containing opinions heard from others without children, and even from some parents.

As the writing flowed, it became very necessary to give a voice to those who cannot have children for reasons other than choice. Further, I am happy to have expanded further outside the realm of the initial idea. Many people have told me they would love to be reading a book solely from the male perspective about life without children. I believe this book has achieved that and gives a little more than what readers will expect.

I give most humble thanks to family, colleagues and friends who supported this project.

I acknowledge the contribution of Robert Kozak, a writer and proud parent, who suggested part of the title, then willingly handed it over to me suggesting it would be a good reflection on what I wanted to say.

I want to express my profound gratitude to the many parents, and non-parents, who encouraged the writing of Planned UnParenthood through social media outlets, e-mails and telephone calls.

I want to acknowledge the many people who have inspired my drive to work in writing. There are so many people that I just cannot list them here. You know who you are, and I humbly thank you.

Finally, I want to thank my wife Cheryl. She has inspired me to speak out, live life to the fullest and pursue my "real" job. Her edits to this book make it all the more enjoyable to read, after making it all the more enjoyable to write.

William (Dann) Alexander

www.ingramcontent.com/pod-product-compliance
Lightning Source LLC
Chambersburg PA
CBHW031505270326
41930CB00006B/256